T0327289

Your Personal Tuning Fork: The Endocrine System

A Way to Sustainable Health ... in a Fragile World

Your Personal Tuning Fork: The Endocrine System

A Way to Sustainable Health ...
in a Fragile World

Deborah K. Bates

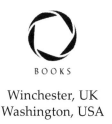

BOOKS

Winchester, UK
Washington, USA

First published by O-Books, 2012
O-Books is an imprint of John Hunt Publishing Ltd., Laurel House, Station Approach,
Alresford, Hants, SO24 9JH, UK
office1@o-books.net
www.o-books.com

For distributor details and how to order please visit the 'Ordering' section on our website.

Text copyright: Deborah K. Bates 2010

ISBN: 978 1 84694 503 8

All rights reserved. Except for brief quotations in critical articles or reviews, no part of
this book may be reproduced in any manner without prior written permission from
the publishers.

The rights of Deborah K. Bates as author have been asserted in accordance with the Copyright,
Designs and Patents Act 1988.

A CIP catalogue record for this book is available from the British Library.

Design: Lee Nash

Printed in the UK by CPI Antony Rowe
Printed in the USA by Offset Paperback Mfrs, Inc

We operate a distinctive and ethical publishing philosophy in all
areas of our business, from our global network of authors to
production and worldwide distribution.

CONTENTS

To those whose pursuit of wellbeing is authentic.

To Charlotte and Colby who by virtue of their desire to have their mother around for a long time inspired me to always seek the highest possible solutions, in particular towards the pursuit of holistic living and wellbeing.

To my brother Darryl ... through his last breath he showed me how to take my next breath.

To Ameliah, Lucas, Connor ... from your Bi Bi.

To Mum and Dad ... you paved the way.

Acknowledgments

I cannot produce this book without appreciation and gratitude for the following people:

Clients — without whom I would not have discovered the journey of self healing.

Jules Watson (author of the Dalriada Trilogy, The Raven Queen and the Swan Maiden) — your words of encouragement inspired me to continue honing my craft. "Be bold! You will only regret not being bold."

Paulo Coelho (most widely read and one of the most influential authors of today) — your message to me, "Nothing is impossible as long as you wish it with all your heart," inspired me to move forward.

Epigraph

["Life has the answers and as a being of life so too we have the answers ..."]

An oriental fable tells of the ancient Gods trying to decide where to hide the power of the universe so that humans would not find it and use it destructively.

'One God said, "Let's hide it on top of the highest mountain."

But they decided that humans would eventually climb the highest mountain and find the great power.

Another God said, "Let's hide the great power at the bottom of the deepest ocean."

Again it was decided that humans would eventually explore the depths of the sea.

The third God suggested, "Let us hide the great power of the universe in the middle of the earth."

But alas, they realized that humans would someday conquer that too.

Finally the wisest God of all said, "I know what to do. Let us hide the great power of the universe within man. He will never think to look for it there!"'

Your Personal Tuning Fork: The Endocrine System is a book about seeking answers and finding them within.

Medical data demonstrates that humans possess great powers within, which most fail to use. These powers estimate that 75 per cent of humans use only 25 per cent of their physical powers. Based on those statistics, we are only half alive. Imagine if we were fully alive — now that's working towards sustainable health!

Preface

The Pursuit

["Life is fragile, and it is through this fragility that we find strength ..."]

For as long as I can recall, I have been in pursuit ... to find meaning, a way of living in a world which seemed precarious. Life is fragile, and it is through this fragility that we find strength, and so it became imperative to me, if I were to live in a precarious world, in fragility, it was necessary for me to discover the source of this strength. This pursuit led me to attain degrees in the study of philosophy, religion, and metaphysics. I was led further into my pursuit through the study of alternative health practices — anything that embraced the spirit and soul with the physical in total wellbeing. I trained as a metaphysical healer in 1995; in 1997 I became a practitioner in Kinesiology and Touch for Health along with Reiki and Bach Flower essences.

As my practice grew, so too awareness grew of a health connection between emotions and the physiological, as clients sought relief from physical symptoms in addition to emotional relief. So in part I became a Counselor and subsequently gained a Diploma (Clinical) in Professional Counseling and Life Coaching in 1998. This led to numerous certificates in genetic blue-printing, relationships, grief and so on. Thus, my academic journey led me through the studies of the human body as a physiological, psychological, philosophical and metaphysical being culminating into an understanding of self-care practices towards holistic wellbeing.

And the pursuit continued ...

The Discovery

["... to live in a precarious world - in fragility, it was necessary to discover the source of this strength ..."]

My career jettisoned forward, and in 1999 I embarked upon a circuit of lectures and discussions. I began to facilitate workshops covering topics from the aura, chakras, color healing and alternative healing techniques, to motivation, goal-setting, personality profiling, blue-printing and personal development. I gave talks for health and wellbeing organizations and groups on these subjects as well as self-care approaches, supplements, stress, and environmental pollutants. The more I spoke with clients (or clients spoke with me) the more a common thread became apparent.

I discovered:

1. They too, were in pursuit, a way of living in a world that seemed precarious — a way of living in health.
2. They all wanted longevity with wellbeing.
3. They were all hungry for answers to everyday health discomforts.
4. They wanted to feel in control of their health, to conduct their own self-care practices.
5. Importantly, I discovered the concept of sustainable health.

And the pursuit had a direction ...

The Link

["... much of our strength — in a fragile and precarious place is found through the application of working as a holistic being ..."]

Yet, it seemed there was something missing. As holistic beings, there had to be a link between the physiological and the subtler energies. And this link would be the key to sustainable health.

So I dug deeper. I searched for a key, a way to link it all together. And I found the key — the link — and this link between the physical, emotional and subtle bodies was a link to sustainable health and it is the endocrine system.

More than a physiological system, this amazing system of glands is a holistic key. Moreover, it is a vital link between the physical body and the subtle energies, embracing all aspects of our existence, emotionally, mentally, physically and spiritually. Thus the endocrine system, as a link, holds the power — it is the key towards sustaining fragility or maintaining strength in a precarious world.

And so I discovered that much of our strength, in a fragile and precarious place, is found through the application of working as a holistic being, supporting all aspects of our existence: emotionally, mentally, physically and spiritually. And the way to holistic sustainable health is via the endocrine system.

And the pursuit had meaning ...

The Story

[*"With all parts cooperating, we stand strong and unified in total wellbeing thus, fragility finds strength."*]

And so ... it all became apparent. The endocrine system, as an amazing system of glands producing life-sustaining hormones and chemicals, was the key towards sustainable health and wellbeing — holistically.

It made sense.

Its story begged to be told.

It made even more sense that this story begged to be presented as a holistic approach to self-care encompassing the subtle body.

The endocrine system is not a physiological system in isolation. For little in life is in isolation and to isolate any part weakens us. With all parts co-operating, working healthily together, we stand strong and unified in total wellbeing, and thus, fragility finds strength.

So I began to tell its story. The more I tuned into its story, the more I saw a correlation between the endocrine system and a tuning fork.

Thus the story — *Your Personal Tuning Fork: The Endocrine System* has earned its place.

And the pursuit found rest …

~

Begin your pursuit …

Make your own discoveries; discover how to keep your system finely tuned for sustainable health. This easy to read, one-stop guide, takes you to the endocrine glands, hormones, stress over-load, chakras, meridians, acupressure points, exercises, symptom repertory, body system charts, complimentary therapies guide, thyroid and chakra self care tests, balancing techniques and daily tuning plans. It will leave you feeling empowered to become your own health-master to take charge of your well-being and life.

Deborah K Bates

Grab your *Personal Tuning Fork* and *'twang'* your way to sustainable health!

"Health (Old Style)"

In that condition the whole body is elevated to a state by others
    unknown —
inwardly and outwardly illuminated,
purified, made solid,
strong, yet buoyant.
A singular charm,
more than beauty,
flickers out of,
and over, the face —
a curious transparency beams in the eyes,
both in the iris and the white —
the temper partakes also ...
... the play of the body in motion takes a previously
unknown grace.
Merely to move is then a happiness,
a pleasure — to breathe, to see, is also.
All the beforehand gratifications,
drink, spirits, coffee,
grease,
stimulants, mixtures,
late hours, luxuries, deeds of the night,
seem as vexatious dreams,
and now the awakening:-
many fall into their natural places,
wholesome,
conveying diviner joys

~ Walt Whitman ~

Introduction

["A key to sustainable health is the Endocrine System: our personal tuning fork."]

Your Personal Tuning Fork: The Endocrine System is a book about health — Sustainable Health.

It Discusses:

- Daily disturbances which interfere with health

- The endocrine system and how it relates to health and health disturbances

- The endocrine system as our personal tuning fork

- The concept of holism or totalism towards sustainable heath

It Takes You on a Tour:

- Of the body via the endocrine system exploring the glands and hormones - and how it tunes the body's systems and organs back into health

- Beyond the physical body into the unique interaction between the physical and the subtle energies known as the meridians and chakras and how integral this relationship is to total well-being

It Demonstrates:

- How to identify imbalances and correct them with natural and safe remedies

- Self-care techniques to assist your journey towards sustainable health

- A how-to-daily-tuning-guide

- Safe and simple practices to maintain a balanced and fluid connection between the physical and subtle bodies

["Allow yourself to gain the understanding and then you will be guided towards a greater sense of wellbeing and harmony."]

Sustainable health is about health as a holism or totalism. It's about understanding that we are whole as an energetic being and herein is a way to sustainable health — and a link is via the endocrine system.

In my practice, it is not uncommon for a client to present with symptoms ranging from emotional, mental to physiological. I have seen a connection, like a thread that weaves or a tuning fork that balances a melody, it is found in the marvel of the endocrine system.

Issues such as loss of libido, depression, mood swings, and inability to lose or gain weight, lethargy, low self esteem, brain fatigue are often raised by clients in our consultations and can often be related to a sluggish link in the endocrine system.

Assisting the client with information regarding their endocrine system equips them with knowledge regarding how their body works and a consequence is empowerment to enhance wellbeing including relationships and daily living. A developed understanding regarding 'the how to' and 'why this is happening' greatly improves the ability to self heal.

How to Use This Book

Your Personal Tuning Fork: The Endocrine System takes you on a journey into the human body, its processes and systems as both a physical and metaphysical being. As a reference piece, its purpose is to acquaint the reader with their own personal tuning fork and to guide regarding the functionality and processes of the endocrine system, with a goal towards self-empowerment through knowledge. It presents safe, simple techniques to enable a creative approach to self-care which engenders greater wellbeing at a holistic level towards sustainable health.

I encourage you to read this book through at least once in its entirety before attempting to make changes. Allow yourself to gain the understanding and then you will be guided towards the most appropriate processes and areas of your body requiring attention. The alternative methods I present in this book are not designed or intended to be a panacea for all health problems. They are not an attempt to turn people away from doctors, medicines, or surgery.

If any of the information provided in this book alerts you to a health concern, I encourage you to seek the opinion of a professional practitioner and follow their suggestions towards greater wellbeing.

~

Your Personal Tuning Fork: The Endocrine System is an easy to read daily reference for every-day solutions to every-day issues.

What is Health …
What is Sustainable Health?

["… to hold up and endure a state of wholeness, being sound or well, holy, sacred.."]

Health is a big word and we expect a lot from it. Most people want to improve their health. We want good health and if we don't have good health we wonder where it is gone. We want it along with longevity. In essence we want sustainable health, something that won't go away.

In terms of achieving sustainable health, I guess it serves to understand what sustainable health is.

The word **health** means, 'wholeness, being whole, sound or well,' and 'holy, sacred.'

The word **sustain** means to 'hold up, endure.'

And so, **sustainable health** is to hold up in endurance as a state of being, whole or well or that which is holy and sacred. Now that's profound!

Longevity, Wellbeing and Those Sneaky Disturbances

["Health should not come and go…what comes and goes is our awareness …"]

Most people want longevity, longevity that is, hand-in-hand with wellbeing. We have the ability to live longer today — to live longer and healthier.

Today, we are privileged to have improved medical processes, interventions and knowledge regarding health and wellbeing yet, the environments we live in have the potential to impact our health adversely, such as toxic chemicals and pollutants. More than that, we live busy lives, cram more into daily regimes, we drink more, eat more, stress more, push the boundaries more, we sleep less, relax less, exercise less, and often we take for granted that our bodies will continue working despite these 'more or less' states.

For most of us, we cast little thought to our bodies, perhaps only thinking about it when illness or disturbance strikes. Disturbances such as allergies, brain fatigue, dizziness, general aches and pains, headaches, insomnia, lethargy, loss of libido, low self-esteem, mood swings, sugar cravings, and weight issues interfere with daily life interrupting sustainable health. And this is when we see that health is something that comes and goes.

But health is not about the absence of disease. Health should not come and go. Health is a state of being and ever-present. What comes and goes is our awareness of it. It is the *little thought to the daily disturbances* that get in *health's way*.

[*"Health should be a dynamic place of being — ever present."*]

If we want longevity with health, it is imperative to understand what that means and how to apply it to our lives.

Health should be a dynamic place of being — ever present — sustainable. The word dynamic means 'powerful, power' and 'to be able to have power.'

And so if health is a dynamic place of being, health is a place of power. It requires the totality of our being to sustain that power. When I talk of the totality of our being, I mean at all levels.

The terms — spiritually, mentally, emotionally, and physically or mind body and soul — have been used and used and used, to the point where they are somewhat of a cliché. Clichés aside, the message is the same. All of the afore-mentioned terms demonstrate a totality or a holism. And holism is about all parts working together, anything in isolation is weakened; this is a law of physics. There will always be strength — power — dynamism in the totally of an entity. Thus for ever-present health, it is paramount to be ever-present, employing the totality of our being, deploying the energies to sustain that ever-present state of health. The state of homeostasis is dependent upon that.

Holism, Totalism and the Body-Thought Connection

["… health requires a totalism of energies to be sustained."]

The subject of holistic health or health in terms of *totalism* goes back in time … way back … and embraces a multitude of practices. The ancient Greeks, Persians, and Hindus felt that every part of the body had a secret meaning and a role to play in wellbeing. History is dotted with theories and examples of how health requires a totalism of energies to be sustained. And how our health is affected by aspects of our being which are out-of-kilter or balance — where homeostasis is interrupted. I call this the *body-thought connection* — our thought/emotional patterns and resultant physiological outcomes.

It has been said that 70% of disease is as a result of emotional repression. The emotions have been linked to the physical body for centuries. Chinese medicine drew correlations between the physical energies of the organs and the emotions centuries ago and they have a sophisticated holistic system of healthcare using the meridians.

Today we are educated with a greater acceptance and awareness between the physical body and the emotions – *hate* poisons the cells and manifests as skin conditions, cancers and acne; *grief* engulfs our lungs and suffocates our breathing; *fear* paralyses and crystallizes fluids into gall stones or kidney stones; *anger* and *rage* boils the blood and sends toxins into the liver and gall-bladder; *anxiety* churns the stomach and congests the flow of elimination; *regret* and *sorrow* strip the cells of the spleen and pancreas, depleting the sweetness of life; *jealousy* and *envy* sears through the veins and hardens the heart; bitterness and judgement freezes our joints creating arthritis and immobility, and *self-reproach* annihilates the spirit and inhibits healing.

Dr Bach the bacteriologist and pathologist is succinct in his theory of healing using the concept of totalism:

> *'This system of healing, which has been Divinely revealed unto us, shows that it is our fears, our cares, our anxieties and such like that open the path to the invasion of illness. Thus by treating our fears, our cares, our worries and so on, we not only free ourselves from our illness, in addition take away our fears and worries, and leave us happier and better in ourselves.'* (With permission Bach Center, excerpt The Twelve Healers and other remedies.)

Dr Bach was an expert in the field of pathology, homeopathy, and vaccines. He embarked upon research into holistic health which led him to the revelation that traditional medicine ignored the whole person. This revelation took him further into the field of homeopathic and the healing properties of plants and flowers and he discovered *that* an individual's emotional state not only affected their wellbeing but reflected the disease. The result was a selection of remedies known as the Bach Flower Remedies which he calls the *Twelve Healers*. These remedies work on the emotional states and when balance is achieved at this level, equilibrium is restored towards healing as a totalism. Bach's way of medicine hinges upon a system of totality in the treatment of disease towards sustainable health.

In a similar vein, Louise Hay, founder of the self-help movement, discussed the connection between the mind and body in her first book, *Heal Your Body* (Hay House, 1976). This book explains how beliefs and ideas about ourselves are often the cause of our emotional problems and physical maladies. As a result of her work many people have learned how to create greater wellness in their bodies, minds, and spirits.

Totalism is a system of holism and sustainable health is

dependent upon it; and this requires awareness and vigilance.

Being Awake — Coming Back to the Place of Dynamic

["A key to sustainable health is through personal intervention at an awareness level."]

To achieve sustainable health we need to be vigilant towards the system of sustainable health, we need to apply the principles of totalism.

Health and wellbeing is about being in touch with oneself mentally, emotionally, physically and spiritually. A key to sustainable health is through personal intervention at an awareness level. Thus, health and wellbeing is dependent upon vigilance.

The word vigilance is French in origins and means wakefulness. I prefer to use wakefulness or vigilance as opposed to the hackneyed word of awareness as its origins are steeped in being cautious or wary. It is my opinion, when discussing such a powerful topic as health, the inference of wary or caution evokes a sense of diminished power whereas the terms vigilance and wakefulness evoke a sense of power or control.

And so, vigilance is paramount and there is much we can do at an intervention level. Through vigilance we can identify minor disturbances and this improves our ability to self-heal.

Deepak Chopra, who began his career as an endocrinologist, later shifted his focus to alternative medicine with a theme that health can be found through a mind-body-spirit integration. In essence his system of healing speaks of unity, integration and holism – health is more than the absence of disease; it is a dynamic state of balance and integration of body, mind, and spirit.

Deepak Chopra's work signals a time of awakening and vigilance or listening to signals from the body — ridding oneself of negative emotions, thus one can improve and sustain health. Through an understanding of the concept of health and the role of the endocrine system we improve our chances of health as a dynamic place of being as a totalism.

~

So what is health? What is sustainable health?

- Health is sacred something to uphold
- Health is a state of being and ever-present
- Health is a dynamic place of being — in totalism
- Health is not the absence of disease or a goal to be reached
- Health should be sustainable because it is sacred, ours and enduring

Your Personal Tuning Fork: The Endocrine System is a key to sustainable health and a dynamic place of wellbeing.

This story of *Your Personal Tuning Fork: The Endocrine System* is presented in three parts:

PART ONE: The Physical Body

Here, we explore *Your Personal Tuning Fork: The Endocrine System* and how it works within the physical body. The human body is complex and intricate, complete with systems, organs, functions and processes vital to existence and wellbeing. This exploration will assist a deeper understanding of how your body works in conjunction with your endocrine system. You will gain insights and how to honor this remarkable system through proactive involvement towards sustainable health.

PART TWO: The Subtle Body

Here, we explore the subtle body, its processes and its link to the physical which is via *Your Personal Tuning Fork: The Endocrine System.* The human being is a chemical-psychological-spiritual-physiological structure and harmonizing the entire being must include an understanding of all of these aspects. Thus, the techniques expressed within this book address the entire being on a holistic level including using intellectual, thinking, imagination and faith.

PART THREE: Putting It All Together

Here, we explore ways of putting it all together to attain the goal of homeostasis. At this stage, you are acquainted with *Your Personal Tuning Fork: The Endocrine System.* You are ready to explore self-care approaches towards a healthy endocrine system and a way of remaining whole in strength, in a precarious world.

PART ONE: THE PHYSICAL BODY

The best six doctors anywhere
And no one can deny it
Are sunshine, water, rest, and air
Exercise and diet.
These six will gladly you attend
If only you are willing
Your mind they'll ease
Your will they'll mend
And charge you not a shilling.

~ Wayne Fields, What the River Knows, 1990 ~

Tuning Fork

["Tuning Fork ... designed to calibrate pitch"]

John Shore invented an instrument which he called a pitch fork in 1711. Now for most, a pitch fork is a three-pronged instrument used to pick up garden matter. Shore's invention bore a very different design. As a metal instrument with a handle and two prongs or tines designed to calibrate pitch, it performed very different functions to that of the garden variety — to avoid confusion he renamed it and it became the Tuning Fork.

The Tuning Fork is a subtle and precise mechanism used to tune instruments and when struck, produces a sound wave of an almost pure tone or fixed pitch. It works on the process of calibration, which is to adjust or regulate restoring harmony and/or pitch.

The Endocrine System as our Personal Tuning Fork is a subtle and precise mechanism used to tune the instrument known as our body. Like Shore's tuning fork, it too works on the process of calibration, to adjust or regulate our instrument (the body) restoring harmony and thus maintaining homeostasis.

["Our Personal Tuning Fork calibrates our body's processes, to maintain homeostasis."]

Just as a tuning fork needs to be cared for and well maintained to ensure correct pitch and calibration, so too our *Personal Tuning Fork: The Endocrine System,* needs to be healthy and well maintained so it can perform its tuning processes towards maintaining homeostasis — thus ensuring total wellbeing of all our body's processes.

We use a tuning fork on our musical instruments to guarantee reliable tones, perfect pitch and harmony. Likewise, we need our

Personal Tuning Fork for perfect pitch and harmony — to calibrate our body's processes, to maintain homeostasis.

Homeostasis

["Our body's holistic wellbeing is dependent upon the homeostatic balance."]

The body has an infinite number of inter-linked processes; some are simple, and some very complex. The processes of equilibrium and homeostasis are some of the most important of these processes. Simply, this means - keeping the internal body environment in a steady state of being - in balance. Homeostasis is the body's ability to keep all functions in their proper balance, to control its energy flow. It is the body's internal wisdom.

Originating from Greek *homeos* — meaning same and *statos* meaning status — homeostasis is the state of being the same and is one of the most remarkable properties of highly complex organisms, such as a healthy human body, or any living creature for that matter.

Our body's holistic wellbeing is dependent upon the homeostatic balance. The *Personal Tuning Fork* is the mechanism used in this process and it needs to be in perfect pitch to maintain homeostasis.

["Daily life — pollutants, chemicals, stresses, interfere with the body's natural ability to maintain a state of homeostasis"]

Nature has the ability to balance itself in a way that allows a steady equilibrium. It constantly adjusts changes and regulates to restore equilibrium using the processes of homeostasis.

Babes are born with a natural tendency towards the state of equilibrium and homeostasis.

When we, as adults are in a state of holistic wellbeing, we can tend towards equilibrium and homeostasis. However, daily life — pollutants, chemicals, stresses, interfere with the body's natural ability to maintain a state of homeostasis. As a result, our health and bodily processes are continually shifting and adapting to our environment and our experience of life.

In this way, the endocrine system continually seeks equilibrium; our *Personal Tuning Fork* continually seeks to calibrate in order to maintain a state of homeostasis.

How Does Homeostasis Work?

["Our body has to find a way to equilibrate ... this is homeostasis."]

All homeostatic mechanisms use negative feedback to maintain a constant value. Negative feedback means that whenever a change occurs in a system, the change automatically causes a corrective mechanism to start, which reverses the original change and brings the system back to normal. This can also mean that the bigger the change the bigger the corrective mechanism. For example, daily we are exposed to changing environmental conditions. A person threatened by the environment — this can be at a physiological (toxic substances, allergic reaction, chemicals etc) or psychological (trauma, grief, shock etc) — prepares for action. The body mobilizes reserves of energy and produces certain hormones such as adrenalin, which prepare it for flight or fight.

Familiar physiological reactions occur in the presence of emotion, danger, or physical effort — the heart beats faster and respiration quickens. The face turns red or pales and the body perspires. The individual may experience shortness of breath, cold sweats, shivering, and trembling legs. These physiological manifestations reflect the efforts of the body to maintain internal equilibrium. Our body has to find a way to equilibrate and it has many mechanisms to maintain equilibrium even when our external environment is changing.

This is a process of homeostasis.

["Without homeostasis we become ill or experience disease or general lack of wellbeing."]

The endocrine system as a personal tuning fork plays a vital role in homeostasis. This is one of the most important functions of the endocrine system and is achieved via the release of hormones. The hormones use the system of negative feedback to regulate the internal environment as a corrective mechanism to achieve homeostasis.

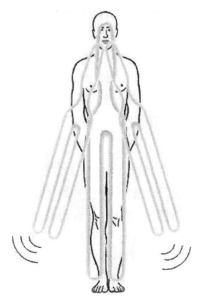

Some examples of homeostasis are found in:

- The regulation of the amount of water and minerals in the body
- The removal of metabolic waste
- The regulation of body temperature
- The regulation of blood glucose level

Homeostasis is imperative because when it fails we become ill or experience disease or general lack of wellbeing.

The Endocrine System

- A control mechanism for the entire body

- The primary goal is to restore homeostasis

- A marvelous system of glands which secrete life sustaining hormones

- Optimizes the functioning of all of the body's processes

["An imbalance in this system can interfere with our ability to sustain health …"]

Complex and finely tuned, the endocrine system acts as a control mechanism for the entire body. It is vital to the coordination of the body's activities and responses to changes in the environment — both internal and external. Without this coordination and unification between the vital centers, the major organs of our being lose their equilibrium and homeostatic state. The consequence can be anything from general lack of wellbeing to more serious conditions which should be treated by a professional.

Of all the body's systems and processes, the endocrine system is the most susceptible to daily stresses, such as thoughts, emotions, environmental factors, nutrition and pollutants. An imbalance in this system can interfere with our ability to sustain health and some of the symptoms can manifest as depression, mood swings, weight or sleep issues, lethargy, low self-esteem, fuzzy brain, loss of libido, headaches, allergies, fatigue, and general aches and pains.

Often we refer to these as little problems or nothing major, yet insidiously they impact our work environment, sleep patterns, relationships, the ability to exercise or eat nutritionally. Loss of libido influences our relationships. Fuzzy thinking influences our ability to work or perform other functions such as driving. Migraines, headaches or pain of any kind influence how we manage our daily lives and routines. Depression clouds our existence and perceptions including how we feel about ourselves. Stress and anxiety influences many areas of our daily lives and influences our behaviors and relationships. These little disturbances can indicate an *out of balance state of being* or an interruption in the homeostatic status. Our *personal* tuning fork has the ability to restore balance and bring about homeostasis.

[*"Disease cannot function in a properly functioning body — a harmonious system ..."*]

The endocrine system acts as a tuning fork and the primary goal is to restore harmonious function so that every part of the whole is doing its work and is in open communication with every other part.

Holistic applications are not about fighting disease, rather, it is about restoring harmonious conditions — homeostasis — and within this environment disease is not tolerated. Disease cannot function in a properly functioning body, a harmonious system, one that does not have its homeostatic state compromised.

It performs this function via a marvelous system of ductless glands. These glands secrete chemical 'messengers' called hormones into the bloodstream which circulate and travel through cells to specific organs. Here they work to optimize functioning of our body's processes such as mood, memory, growth and development, tissue function, metabolism, sexual function and reproduction processes including fertility and pregnancy, hair and bone growth, breast milk production as well as some aspects of personality and behavior.

Endocrine Glands

["… the endocrine glands the invisible guardians …"]

The Rosicrucians named the endocrine glands 'the invisible guardians or the controllers and guardians of life who determine the equilibrium of spiritual and physical forces in mankind.' And to this end, endocrine glands indeed, activate, nourish and support the human form towards sustainable health.

Endocrine glands are ductless life centers, which produce and secrete chemicals into the circulatory system for transport to a target organ. These chemicals and secretions are known as hormones. Releasing more than 20 major hormones directly into the bloodstream, they are transported to cells in other parts of the body. Some glands release their hormones directly into specific areas whilst others select and remove materials from the blood, process them, and then release the finished chemical product for use by the body.

The endocrine glands are:

- Hypothalamus
- Pineal
- Pituitary
- Thyroid
- Para-thyroid
- Thymus
- Pancreas
- Adrenals
- Gonads

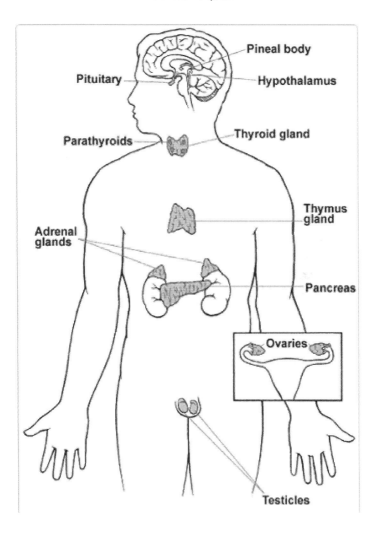

Hormones

["Hormones ... a chemical released from a gland .... A life sustaining fluid"]

In the 1890s, scientists suggested that certain organs of the human body secreted fluids that influenced many of the body's processes. English physiologist Ernest Henry Starling named these fluids after the Greek word *hormone* meaning that which sets in motion or to arouse.

Back then, little was known regarding hormones, today however, we are armed with signification data and scientific information with regard to these life-sustaining fluids.

Simply, hormones act as the body's chemical messengers transferring information and instructions from one set of cells to another. Although many different hormones move through the bloodstream, each type is designed to target certain cells. The rate of production of hormones is regulated by the optimum functioning of the glands associated and a homeostatic control system — the endocrine system.

Influence

In a homeostatic environment, the hormones secreted have an influence upon almost every cell, organ, and function of our bodies.

- They induce a sense of drowsiness that allows a good night's sleep
- They provide extra blood to the muscles for that extra mile
- They speed the fire of passion and warms the libido
- They shower the darkness of the soul with light
- They allow us to make the life-saving leap — just in the nick of time

Chemical Structure

Chemically, hormones fall into three classes and are classified by chemical structure, not function.

1. Steroid hormones (lipids and phospholipids)
Derived from cholesterol. Examples of steroid hormones are testosterone and cortisol. They are secreted by the gonads, adrenal cortex, and placenta.

Lipid and phospholipid derived hormones derive from lipids such as linoleic acid and arachidonic acid and phospholipids.

2. Amino acid derivatives
Derivatives of the amino acids tyrosine and tryptophan. Examples are catecholamines and thyroxine. Amines are derived from the amino acid tyrosine and are secreted from the thyroid and the adrenal medulla.

3. Peptide hormones (poly-peptides)
Peptide and poly-peptides are short chains of amino acids; most hormones are peptides. They are secreted by the pituitary, parathyroid, heart, stomach, liver, and kidneys. Peptides composed of scores or hundreds of amino acids are referred to as proteins. Examples of protein hormones include insulin and growth hormone. More complex protein hormones are carbohydrate side chains and are called glycoprotein hormones. Luteinizing hormone, follicle-stimulating hormone and thyroid-stimulating hormone are glycoprotein hormones.

Functions

Hormones have a multitude of functions and fall into seven

broad areas:

1. Fluidity
   To regulate the chemical composition of the fluid that bathes all of our body's cells and tissues

2. Energy
   Helps to regulate general metabolism and energy balance

3. Regulation
   Assists in the regulation of cardiac and smooth muscle contraction

4. Balance
   Keeps the body in balance in spite of disruptions such as infection, trauma, emotional stress, dehydration, starvation, hemorrhage and temperature extremes

5. Modulation
   Modulates various facets of the immune system

6. Reproducing
   Plays a role in reproduction

7. Supports
   Supports growth and development

Table 1 - Glands, Function, Hormone, Chemical

Hypothalamus Gland

Function   Activates and controls the part of the nervous system that controls involuntary body functions, the hormonal system, and many body functions, such as regulating sleep and stimulating appetite.

Hormone	
Corticotropin-releasing hormone	Polypeptide
Growth hormone-releasing	Polypeptide
Thyrotropin-releasing hormone	Polypeptide
Follicle-stimulating hormone	Polypeptide
Gonadotropin-releasing	Polypeptide
Prolactin-inhibiting factor	Polypeptide
Somatostatin	Polypeptide
Gastrointestinal neuropeptide	Polypeptide
Dopamine	Steroid
Antidiuretic hormone	Polypeptide
Oxytocin	Polypeptide

Pineal Gland

Function   Involved with daily biological cycles

Hormone   Melatonin   Amine

Pituitary gland - Anterior lobe

Function   Produces a number of different hormones that influence various other endocrine glands.

Hormone		
	Corticotropin	Polypeptide
	Growth hormone	Protein
	Thyrotropin thyroid-stimulating	Glycoprotein
	Follicle-stimulating hormone	Glycoprotein
	Lueinizing, cell stimulating	Glycoprotein
	Prolactin	Protein

Pituitary gland - Posterior lobe

Function Produces a number of different hormones that influence various other endocrine glands.

Hormone		
	Oxytocin	Polypeptide
	Vasopressin, antidiuretic hormone	Polypeptide

Thyroid gland

Function Produces hormones that stimulate body heat production, bone growth, and the body's metabolism.

Hormone		
	Thyroxine	Amino acid
	Triiodothyronine	Amino acid
	Calcitonin	Polypeptide

Parathyroid gland

Function Secrete a hormone that maintains the calcium level in the blood.

Hormone		
	Parathyroid hormone	Polypeptide
	Calcitonin	Polypeptide

Thymus

Function   Plays a role in the body's immune
system.

Hormone   Thymosin   Polypeptide

Pancreatic islets

Function   Secretes a hormone (insulin) which
controls the use of glucose by the
body.

Hormone   Glucagon   Polypeptide
Insulin   Polypeptide
Somatostatin   Polypeptide
Pancreatic   Polypeptide

Adrenal gland - Cortex

Function   Performs two functions. One: secrete
hormones that influence the body's
metabolism, blood chemicals, and
body characteristics. Two:
influences the part of the nervous
system involved in the response
and defense actions against stress.

Hormone   Cortisol   Steroid
Corticosterone   Steroid
Aldosterone   Steroid
Androgens   Steroid
Estrogens   Steroid

Adrenal gland - Medulla

Function   Performs two functions. One: secrete hormones that influence the body's metabolism, blood chemicals, and body characteristics. Two: influences the part of the nervous system involved in the response and defense actions against stress.

Hormone	Adrenaline	Amine
	Noreadrenaline	Amine
	Dopamine	Steroid

Testis

Function   Secrete hormones that influence female and male characteristics, respectively.

| **Hormone** | Testosterone | Steroid |

Ovary

Function   Secrete hormones that influence female and male characteristics, respectively.

Hormone	Estrogens	Steroid
	Inhibin	Polypeptide
	Progesterone	Steroid
	Relaxin	Polypeptide

Personal Tuning Fork
— the Individual Glands

- **Hypothalamus**
- **Pineal**
- **Pituitary**
- **Thyroid**
- **Para-thyroid**
- **Thymus**
- **Pancreas**
- **Adrenals**
- **Gonads**

Hypothalamus

(Pronounced: hi-po-tha-luh-mus)

["The Hypothalamus ... its primary function is to regulate homeostasis"]

Some do not consider the hypothalamus to be a true endocrine gland yet its role is quite significant to the function of the endocrine system. Situated in the brain beneath the thalamus, it consists of many aggregations of nerve cells and controls a variety of autonomic functions aimed at maintaining homeostasis.

The hypothalamus sends two hormones, growth hormone (GH) and growth hormone releasing hormone (GHRH) to the pituitary gland. It also governs the body's acid/alkaline balance, makes us sweat if it's hot, keeps us breathing regularly, and controls the part of the nervous system that regulates involuntary muscles. It forms the limbic system which is the seat of emotions, influences digestion, and the rate of respiration in emotional situations. It also regulates the blood to the various organs and is associated with the adrenals in the 'flight or fight' situation.

Together with the pineal and pituitary glands, the hypothalamus forms part of the communication center combining visual, auditory, speech and learning approaches. When heightened, many of the higher intellectual capabilities manifest themselves. Imbalanced function can lead to impairments in verbal ability such as dyslexia, stuttering and inability to think clearly as well as lack of interest and forgetfulness.

Hypothalamus and Weight
Like the pineal gland, the hypothalamus plays an important role in hunger, thirst, sodium levels and salt cravings experienced from time to time along with our electrolyte balance. When our fluid systems are out of whack the hypothalamus signals a need for electrolytes or water.

Have you experienced moments of insatiable, inexplicable thirst? And no matter how much you drink it just doesn't seem enough. These experiences can signal an interruption to the function of the hypothalamus.

As the weight-body-guard, it signals a level of satiety (feeling of fullness) we feel after eating or conversely, the next time you hear your tummy growl the hypothalamus is sending a message that the body needs fuel.

When our hypothalamus is working at optimum levels, our system of sodium and electrolyte levels are functioning at their best to regulate weight, hunger and thirst.

Symptom Repertory:

Physiological	Emotional/Mental
Craving for sodium	Apathy
Dyslexia	Easily confused

Electrolyte imbalance

Excessive appetite or thirst

Forgetfulness

Hypochondria

Impaired speech

Impaired vision

Menstrual irregularities

Not feeling full after eating

Over-weight

Stuttering

Inability to think clearly

Mood Swings

Over Sensitivity

Rigid thoughts

Natural Corrective Measures

- Maintain acid/alkaline balance within the body

- Take regular breaks from computers, televisions and artificial lighting

- Avoid bright light at night, for example, watching TV in bed

- Reduce exposure to electromagnetic fields, such as electric blankets

- Sleep in complete darkness so your body produces more melatonin. For instance, your bedside clock might emit too much light

- Drink plenty of water

- Eat slowly — it takes about 20 minutes for the brain to register that the stomach is full.

NB refer to Part Three — Putting it All Together — *Herbs and Foods for Healthy Endocrine.*

Pineal

(pronounced: pih-nee-ul)

["The Pineal … its primary function is to regulate the body's circadian rhythms"]

The size of a pea, the pineal gland lies immediately beneath the hypothalamus in a tiny cave at the center of the brain. As the last endocrine gland discovered, it was once shrouded in myth, superstition and metaphysical theories.

Supernatural Powers

Philosophers and spiritual adepts have long contemplated the function of the pineal. The ancient Greeks believed it was our connection to the "realms of thought," while French philosopher Renee Descartes referred to it as "the seat of the human soul". Ancient Greek physician Galen of Pergamum (131-201AD) said the pineal was a regulator of thought, and that the soul was anchored there.

Most mystical traditions and esoteric schools have thought this area in the center of the brain, to be the connecting link between the physical and spiritual worlds. Many consider it a powerful source of ethereal energy initiating supernatural powers. Associated with the crown chakra, the hormones released by this gland play a part in the stimulation of the higher-mind and the development of intellectual pursuits. It is said toxins in this gland indicate the spirit is weak due to lack of will combined with an invasion of the psyche.

Function

On a physiological level, the pineal gland is activated by light and works in harmony with the hypothalamus gland directing the body's thirst, hunger, sexual desire and biological clock, which determines how we age. As famous psychic Edgar Cayce (1877-1945) once said: "Keep the pineal gland operating and you won't grow old — you will always be young."

Producing the hormone melatonin (a brain chemical that regulates our sleep rhythms) and trace amounts of the psychedelic chemical dimethyltryptamine similar to the neurotransmitter serotonin, the pineal gland controls sleep-wake rhythms, signals the reproductive system to set a child's birth in motion, and moderates the states of euphoria and depression.

Melatonin is an antioxidant that scavenges free radicals and is important for the regulation of many immune hormones in the body. Just like its cousins, DHEA and coenzyme Q10, melatonin levels deplete as we age. With this decrease there is also a corresponding decline in immune resistance. This suggests that melatonin may play a vital role in disease prevention.

When the pineal is stimulated and functioning optimally, it helps us to sleep and relax, improves the immune system, evokes a natural state of euphoria and higher states of intellect (possibly even visions), and helps alleviate depression and the ageing process.

Light Deprivation and Melatonin

An imbalance of melatonin interferes with the body's circadian rhythms (day/night cycle) and results in light deprivation disorders such as depression, oversleeping, weight gain, fatigue and sadness. Our lifestyles can contribute to a reduction of melatonin. Most of us spend the majority of our day working indoors with little natural light, rush home to spend more time indoors to read, watch television, use the computer, or listen to music. While these are great activities for relaxation, they can deprive us of adequate light to produce healthy melatonin levels. Other factors which can decrease melatonin levels include a high protein diet, overeating, high frequency electromagnetic radiation like computers and power lines, chronic stress, alcohol, tobacco, caffeine, poor sleep and sleeping in a room that emits too much light.

The following symptoms indicate light melatonin deprivation:

- Carbohydrate cravings
- Depression
- Difficulty concentrating
- Irritability
- Low energy
- Reduced libido
- Social withdrawal
- Trouble sleeping
- Weight gain

Other Functions

Along with the hypothalamus, the pineal gland forms part of the brain's communication center, including visual, auditory, speech and learning functions. Imbalanced function can lead to dyslexia, stuttering, forgetfulness and inability to think clearly.

Other pineal secretions stimulate activity in the adrenal glands (the stress response glands that sit on top of the kidneys). Here, the pineal stimulates the adrenals to reabsorb sodium and eliminate excess potassium and control the adrenal's fear response.

The pineal also takes up excess iodine as a backup for the thyroid gland, an important energy and hormonal regulator in the throat.

Symptoms of an Underactive Pineal

Environmental stressors affect pineal function, affecting overall body alertness, temperature levels and hormone operation. These can include unusual light and dark patterns, radiation, magnetic fields, nutritional imbalances such as excessive alcohol and caffeine, temperature swings, and overall daily stress patterns.

Symptom Repertory:

Physiological

Dyslexia
Epilepsy
Glaucoma
Headaches
Hypertension
Irregular sleeping patterns
Lack of interest in present
    moment
Menstrual irregularities
Right eye
SAD or seasonal affective
    disorder
Sodium or potassium
    imbalance
Tendency to worry
    excessively

Emotional/Mental

Hypochondria
Inability to think clearly
Irrational fear of the unknown
Mental disorientation
Mood swings
Nightmares/over-vivid dreams
Paranoia or fanaticism

Natural Corrective Measures

- Stress management techniques such as relaxation

- Twenty minutes of meditation daily can help to raise melatonin levels within the body

- Daily doses of natural light

- Eat foods high in potassium such as brown rice, avocado, broccoli and banana

- Take regular breaks from computers, televisions and artificial lighting

- Avoid bright light at night, for example, watching TV in bed

- Reduce exposure to electromagnetic fields, such as electric blankets

- Sleep in complete darkness so your body produces more melatonin. For instance, your bedside clock might emit too much light

- Avoid use of melatonin-lowering substances such as caffeine, tobacco, alcohol

- Tratak meditation (also known as candle gazing) can stimulate the pineal gland and help produce higher levels of melatonin. As a daily practice, light a candle and use the candle flame to focus the eyes

NB refer to Part Three — Putting it All Together — *Herbs and Foods for Healthy Endocrine.*

Pituitary

(pronounced: puh-**too**-uh-ter-ee)

> [*"The Pituitary ... its primary function is to stimulate growth and cell production"*]

The pituitary gland, although not much bigger than a pea has a huge reputation and is hailed as a master. Located in a small bony cavity behind the root of the nose, it is linked to the hypothalamus via a small stalk at the base of the brain.

Often referred to as the third eye possessing mystical powers it is known to contain a complete map of the visual field of the eyes. It plays a major role as a receiver and transformer of universal and vibratory signals and then sends messages so that the rest of the body can respond and adjust.

Master Gland

The pituitary gland is considered the most important part of the endocrine system and is often called the master gland because it makes hormones that control several other endocrine glands. For example — the thyroid hormone is made upon the pituitary's request. It is then released into the body in the form of thyrotrophic hormone.

Like a music conductor orchestrating his orchestra the pituitary directs our personal aria. Because the pituitary seeks to balance the endocrine orchestra any troubles here and in the pineal area, affect the function of the entire body. When changes produce imbalances, the pituitary secretes a hormone to stimulate the under-active glands to restore balance.

The tiny pituitary is divided into two parts: the *anterior lobe* and the *posterior lobe*.

Anterior Lobe

The anterior lobe regulates the activity of the thyroid, adrenals, and reproductive glands.

Pituitary anterior lobe produces the following hormones:

- Growth hormone — stimulates the growth of bone and other body tissues and plays a role in the body's handling of nutrients and minerals.

- Prolactin — activates milk production in women who are breastfeeding.

- Thyrotropin — stimulates the thyroid gland to produce thyroid hormones.

- Corticotropin — stimulates the adrenal gland to produce certain hormones.

Posterior Lobe

The posterior lobe makes and releases the anti-diuretic hormone which helps control body water balance through its effect on the kidneys and urine output.

Function

The pituitary also secretes endorphins, chemicals that act on the nervous system to reduce sensitivity to pain. In addition, the pituitary secretes hormones that signal the ovaries and testes to make sex hormones, controls ovulation and the menstrual cycle in women. The production and secretion of pituitary hormones can be influenced by factors such as emotions and seasonal changes. For example stress switches this gland off, as does the over-use of sunglasses, televisions, computers and fluorescent lights. The pituitary needs sunlight for optimal functioning.

As with the hypothalamus and the pineal, the pituitary gland form part of the communication center and combine visual, auditory, speech and learning approaches. When heightened, many of the higher intellectual capabilities manifest themselves. Imbalanced function can lead to impairments in dyslexia, stuttering and inability to think clearly as well as lack of interest and forgetfulness. Exhaustion in the pituitary function can weaken the sex drive.

Symptom Repertory:

Physiological	Emotional/Mental
Abnormal blood cholesterol	Fanatical thinking
Decreased muscle mass	Fuzzy brain
Decreased stamina and	Mood swings
exercise ability	Loss of libido
Excessive urination/	Rigid thinking
incontinence or	
bed-wetting	
Fat deposits on the hips,	
thighs, chest or abdomen	
Fatigue	
Frontal headaches	
Giantism or Dwarfism	
High blood pressure	
Imbalances in the thyroid,	
pancreas, adrenals,	
liver and kidneys	
Left eye	
Low tolerance for pain	
Sensitivity to light	

Two Self-tests to Check Pituitary Health:

ONE: You will need a small torchlight and the assistance of another person we will call the tester.

1. Close your eyes.

2. Hold your right arm relaxed at your side and left arm held straight out, parallel to the floor. (Either arm can be used for testing. If one side becomes fatigued, the other can be used.)

3. The tester will face you and place their left hand on your right shoulder to steady you. With their right hand, they will grasp your extended arm just above the wrist.

4. Have your tester hold the torchlight onto the area between the eyes in the middle of the brow.

5. The tester will switch the torchlight on and push down on your arm whilst you attempt to resist. (They will push down on the arm firmly, just hard enough to feel the spring and bounce in the arm.)

6. If your arm does not test strong, (i.e. the arm weakens to the pressure) this will indicate a sluggish pituitary, pineal or hypothalamus gland.

TWO: Another test for the pituitary is through observation when moving from a darkened environment to a light or sunny environment. If your eyes find discomfort adjusting to the light this could indicate a sluggish pituitary, pineal or hypothalamus gland.

[Note: these tests are designed for self-care management; they are not designed to take the role of your professional health practitioner.]

Natural Corrective Measures

- Color therapy, it is believed when the energy of color enters our body, it stimulates two of our major glands, the pituitary and pineal glands. This affects the production of various hormones, which in turn affects a variety of physiological and metabolic processes

- Massage the third eye area, located in the slight indent between the eyes on the forehead. Massage upward and outward in a half-inch radius for 30 seconds

- Tratak meditation (also known as candle gazing) can stimulate the pituitary gland and help produce higher levels of melatonin. As a daily practice, light a candle and use the candle flame to focus the eyes

- Brahmari (Humming Bee) Breathing. Place the index finger and middle finger on the area between the eyes and just above the bridge of the nose. Sit comfortably, relax and close the eyes. Begin to hum like a bee on the long outward breath. As you hum you will notice a vibration in the bones of our head. If the hum is low you will feel it more in the jaw whereas a higher hum brings the vibration up into the cheek bones and forehead. This higher humming is said to be very beneficial for the pituitary gland.

NB refer to Part Three — Putting it All Together — *Herbs and Foods for Healthy Endocrine.*

Thyroid

(pronounced: thigh-royd)

["The Thyroid ... its primary function is to regulate the body's metabolism"]

The thyroid gland is the biggest gland in the neck. Situated in the anterior neck below the skin and muscle layers, it has two wings much like a butterfly which wrap around the trachea.

Function

The primary function of the thyroid is to regulate the body's metabolism. It tells the body's cells to burn the amount of food necessary and to produce the amount of energy needed to maintain the body at the required temperature. It does this by producing the hormones thyroxine, triiodothyronine and calcitonin, which stimulate metabolism, body heat production and bone growth. This is usually upon the specific request of the pituitary. These hormones are necessary for maintaining equilibrium in the body and they go directly to the target cells which control metabolic rate. When thyroxine falls below a certain level the brain sends a message via the pineal to the pituitary to produce more.

The hormones released by the thyroid influence nerve stability and proper nerve activity in addition to heart function, respiration and blood pressure. It is documented that the entire blood supply passes through the thyroid gland every 17 minutes. As a result the bloodstream becomes charged with the energy packed secretions designed to lessen nervous tension and induce restful sleep.

As there are two lobes associated with the thyroid, attention should be focused on left and right balance, and whether both or one are hypo or hyperactive. Problems here affect the function of basic metabolism, speed of digestion, nutrient assimilation, weight, warmth etc. The throat is the area of voice expression, and is easily affected by either excessive expression or repression of strong emotions. Exhaustion in the thyroid function can weaken the sex drive. Thyroid function is affected by poor circulation, as it takes longer for hormones to reach areas of repair.

Common Thyroid Problems

The thyroid gland is prone to several very distinct problems, some of which are extremely common. These problems can be broken down into those concerning the production of too much or too little hormone.

Too Much Hormone

Goiter

Thyroid goiter is a dramatic enlargement of the thyroid gland causing compression of important neck structures or simply appearing as a mass in the neck.

Goiters are often removed because of cosmetic reasons or, more commonly, because they compress other vital structures of the neck, including the trachea and the esophagus making breathing and swallowing difficult. Although rare, goiters can grow into the chest. Goiters are usually caused by insufficient iodine in the diet.

Symptom Repertory Goiter:

Physiological	Emotional/Mental
Swelling of the thyroid gland in the neck	Emotional upsets
Diminished power of concentration	Irritability

Swallowing problems, if the goiter is large enough to press on the esophagus
Hyperactivity

Breathing problems, if the goiter is large enough to press on the windpipe (trachea)
Restlessness

Hyperthyroidism

Hyperthyroidism means too much thyroid hormone, the thyroid is considered over-active. Current methods used for treating a hyperthyroid patient are radioactive iodine, anti-thyroid drugs, or surgery. Each method has advantages and disadvantages and are selected for individual patients.

Symptom Repertory High Thyroid Function — Over-active:

Physiological
Addictions
Anxiety
Bulging eyes
Diarrhea
Excessive sweating
Eye/vision changes
Hair loss
Hyperactivity
Increased appetite
Insomnia
Jittery movements
Rapid heart beat/palpitations
Rapid weight loss

Emotional/Mental
Impatience
Inability to focus on one thing
Irritability
Mood Swings
Restlessness
Scattered disconnected thoughts

Too Little Hormone

Hypothyroidism

Hypothyroidism means too little thyroid hormone, the thyroid is considered under-active. If insufficient iodine is supplied not enough thyroxine will be produced and the body produces too little thyroid hormone. The rate of metabolism slows causing mental and physical sluggishness. A decreased activity of the thyroid gland may affect all body functions.

Hypothyroidism can be caused by a problem with the thyroid itself, (primary) or by the malfunction of the pituitary gland or hypothalamus (secondary). This condition is often present for a number of years before it is recognized and treated.

Primary — Thyroid can't produce the amount of hormones requested by the pituitary. The pituitary is requesting hormone release but the thyroid can't produce them.

Secondary — Thyroid can't produce hormones, the pituitary is not stimulating the thyroid to produce hormones.

Acidity and Hypothyroidism

One problem with hypothyroidism is that it is sometimes missed in diagnosis. Even if you haven't been diagnosed with Hypothyroidism, it is important to check your body's overall PH balance for high acidity.

Accumulation of acids in the body due to insufficient digestion of food, food allergies, high intake of acid forming foods and substances can depress the thyroid function. This can also include exposure to heavy metals and toxic chemicals in water and highly processed foods. When the acid levels in the body rise too high, the thyroid becomes depressed and metabolism slows and generates sluggishness in all the body's systems.

With a depressed thyroid function, the body's cells and organs will not metabolize as quickly as they should. The excess acid only serves to make the problem worse and the thyroid will struggle to assist the body to eliminate the acid build up. This only serves to perpetuate the state of Hypothyroidism and impairs digestive processes, reduces immune function, reduces intake of glucose and oxygen into the bloodstream and depletes the body of nutrients integral for wellbeing. And the cycle perpetuates.

Hypothyroidism can cause many degenerative diseases. A functioning thyroid can restore balance and overall health. By neutralizing the acids in the body and eliminating the acid-forming substances from the diet gives the thyroid a chance to heal.

Once you have checked your acid levels, if they are high, take dietary steps to reduce acid levels. (see chapter 'High on Acid' in 'Putting it Altogether'). As acid levels fall the thyroid function will increase.

Symptom Repertory of Low Thyroid Function — Under-active:

Physiological
Back pain
Brittle hair and nails
Cold hands and feet
Constipation
Digestive problems
Droopy eyelids
Dry or itchy skin
Fatigue
Frequent infections
Headaches
Heavy menstrual bleeding
    PMS
Increased cholesterol levels
Infertility/repeated

Emotional/Mental
Anxiety
Apathy
Depression
Lack of motivation
Sluggish thoughts
Teary
Unexplained fears

  miscarriages
Loss of libido
Low basal temperature
    (below 97.8)
Low pulse rate
Poor memory or concentration
Puffiness around face and neck
Shortness of breath
Sleep disorders
Swelling of the legs
Vague aches and pains
Weight gain or inability to lose
    weight

Two Easy Self-care Tests

If you suspect a sluggish thyroid, the following two thyroid function tests can be easily performed at home as part of your self care program. Remember, these tests are not meant to diagnose low or high thyroid conditions, they simply confirm a sluggish thyroid. You can choose whether to pursue medical testing if you are concerned.

Basal Metabolic Rate (BMR) Temperature Test

It is well documented thyroid blood tests can be inaccurate tools for diagnosis because there is such a fine line between a normally functioning thyroid and one that is under active or sluggish. A solution used by many holistic doctors, is taking your underarm temperature before rising in the morning.

Dr Barnes developed the Barnes Basal Temperature Test for thyroid function in 1942. It relies on a morning, waking, underarm temperature, which Dr Barnes believes should average 97.8 to 98.2 (36.6C and 36.8C), to indicate normal thyroid function. Dr Barnes considers temperatures below 97.8 a possible sign of low thyroid function.

Barnes Basal Temperature Test

If using a regular thermometer, shake down the thermometer the night before.

First thing in the morning before rising, place the thermometer under your left armpit for 60 seconds until the thermometer is ready or if digital, beeps.

Record the temperature on a calendar or a chart and continue every day for a month.

In general, the normal temperature range is between 97.8 F and 98.2 F (36.6C and 36.8C). If you find that your readings are consistently and significantly below or above this range, it is a good indicator that you may have compromised thyroid function. Make an appointment to see a natural/holistic or medical doctor for further testing.

Menstruating women should take the test beginning on the second day of menstruation because that is when the body temperature is the lowest.

Take an average of five days' readings.

Iodine Test

Here is an easy way to see if you are iodine deficient:

Rub a dark, orange circle of tinctured iodine (available at most health food stores and pharmacies) on your lower abdomen.

Check the circle every two hours to see if it is still there and note when it begins to fade or disappear.

If your body has sufficient iodine reserves, the circle should stay dark for 24 hours. If the patch fades or disappears quickly it may be because it is being absorbed, indicating that you may be deficient in iodine which may affect proper thyroid function.

[Note: these tests are designed for self-care management; they are not designed to take the role of your professional health practitioner.]

Natural Corrective Measures

- Intake of foods high in iodine such as kelp.

- Gentle tapping of the thyroid gland. (Locate the area where you would find the adams-apple on the trachea)

- Balance PH levels.

NB refer to Part Three — Putting it All Together — *Herbs and Foods for Healthy Endocrine.*

Parathyroid

["The Parathyroid ... its primary function is to regulate the calcium level in the blood"]

Parathyroid glands are four tiny glands the size and shape of a grain of rice, located behind the thyroid. Although they are neighbors and form part of the endocrine system, the thyroid and parathyroid glands are otherwise unrelated.

Function
The primary purpose of the parathyroid gland is to regulate the calcium levels in the blood to a very narrow range ensuring optimum function of the nervous and muscular systems. In this way, the parathyroid's control the levels of calcium in the bones as well as bone strength and density. Other parathyroid functions are the regulation of phosphorus in the body, and giving the spleen advance warning of any foreign substance absorbed by the mouth.

When calcium is deficient in the diet the parathyroid glands leech it from the bones, this creates the condition of osteoporosis. Conversely, if there is an over-activity of one or more the glands, it makes too much hormone, causing a potentially serious calcium imbalance called hyperparathyroidism.

When calcium levels drop below normal, this can be felt as tingling sensations or cramps in the fingers or hands.

Symptom Repertory:

Physiological

Allergies
Arthritis
Back pain
Brittle bones
Calcium or Phosphorous
    deficiency
Gastric/peptic ulcers
High blood pressure
High cholesterol
Irregular sleeping patterns
Kidney stones
Muscle twitching
Muscular cramps
Osteoporosis
Run-down
Tingling in hands and feet
Tooth decay

Emotional/Mental

Foggy head
Irritability
Nervous stress
Poor memory

Natural Corrective Measures

- A deficiency in calcium is not an indicator that the parathyroid is under-functioning

- If Vitamin D levels are low, the intestines have a hard time absorbing calcium

NB refer to Part Three: Putting it All Together — *Herbs and Foods for Healthy Endocrine.*

Thymus

["The Thymus ... its primary function is to rebalance our life energy"]

The word thymus is derived from the Greek *thymos* which denotes life force, soul, and feeling or sensibility. Even the earliest origins of the word implied rising up into flames, as a cloud th spirit.

No one knew much about the thymus until recently. We are just now unraveling the mysteries of this gland. During autopsies it was noticed that young adults who had died in traumatic accidents often had much larger thymus glands than those dying from diseases of a chronic nature. It was also believed that the thymus ceased to function or atrophied after childhood. As a valuable part of the body's immune system, it is controversial as to whether this is true or not.

A pink-grey organ, the thymus gland lies underneath the top of the breast bone. It is the controller of energy flow to the body. Day after day, moment by moment, it monitors and rebalances our life energy. Everything affects the thymus — food, posture, emotional attitudes, stress, physical environment, and social environment. As it is involved with the strength of muscular contraction, muscular weakness can be a symptom of an under-active thymus.

T-cells

T-cells, (T-lymphocytes, a type of white blood cell) play a signif-icant and essential role in immunity and body defence, and is integral to the flow of lymph throughout the body. The thymus acts as emissary to the lymphatic system and secretes thymosin hormone which enhances T-cell performance.

Produced early in life, T-cells are vital to the protection of the immune system, without which we lack resistance to infections, invading bacteria, virus, abnormal cell growth such as cancer and identifying foreign bodies.

Extensive research and experiments have been performed in relation to the thymus and cures for cancer or immunological diseases. One such study experimented on animals where they had their thymus removed and developed cancer rapidly upon injection of cancer cells into their body, while animals with an intact thymus would in most cases react by destroying the cancer cells.

Because this gland is near the heart chakra, it reflects both the positive and negative condition of love and its attributes of enthusiasm, warmth, generosity or conversely, selfishness, apathy, and inability to love. The thymus is said to function better in a loving person and is also programmed to inhibit the sex glands while children are maturing thus enabling the child to demonstrate and develop non-sexual expressions of love and warmth.

Symptom Repertory:

Physiological	Emotional/Mental
Allergies	Irritability
Chemical sensitivities	Mental disorientation
Extreme sweating	Over-reaction to stress
Fatigue	
Lack of general wellbeing	
Lowered Immune	
Muscular weakness	
Puffiness of the throat	
Reacting to chemicals in an unexpected manner, such as drinking caffeine and then being able to sleep easily	
Swollen glands	
Toxicity	

Natural Corrective Measures

- Tapping the thymus gland (the area just below the hollow in the neck below the trachea) throughout the day will kick-start it.

- Acupuncture enhances many immune functions and may increase the number of lymphocytes including T cells, B cells and natural killer cells.

- The most important factor that stimulates and supports our body's immune function is a positive and balanced emotional state. This can be attained through a number of methods including playing with pets or children, laughing, having fun, doing what you love, skilled relaxation, positive affirmations, visualizations or imagery, nurturing yourself, getting adequate rest and exercise, achieving goals and enjoying life.

- Avoid foods rich in sugar, white flour products, artificial and processed foods, saturated fats, caffeine, nicotine, excessive red meat intake and full fat dairy products.

- Living in clean environments with good fresh air circulation is important to health.

- The immune system is greatly influenced by regular exercise. Two great forms of exercise for the lymphatic system are skipping and bouncing daily on a mini trampoline.

- Regular detoxification increases immune response, gives the immune system a chance to repair, heals damage and prolongs life. Fasting rapidly builds lost energy levels and restores vital organ function.

- Homeopathy can be used effectively in the treatment of immune depression and emotional rebalancing.

- Laughter has an anti-stress effect on the body. It can lower serum cortisol and adrenaline, ease the body's stress response and preserve immune function. Smile and laugh more often.

NB refer to Part Three: Putting it All Together — *Herbs and Foods for Healthy Endocrine.*

Pancreas

["The Thymus … its primary function is to regulate sugars into the bloodstream"]

The pancreas is an amazing organ and approximately 5 percent of the total pancreatic mass is comprised of endocrine cells. These cells are clustered in groups within the pancreas and look like little islands of cells. Hence, the familiar name is Islets of Langerhan and these pancreatic islets have two main functions: [1] to produce pancreatic endocrine hormones (e.g. insulin and glucagon) which help regulate many aspects of our metabolism, and [2] to produce pancreatic digestive enzymes.

Insulin Hormone

The insulin hormone is responsible for the transferring of amino acids and fatty acids, together with glucose from the bloodstream, into the cell structure. Simply, it keeps sugar levels from getting too high by converting sugar in the blood to glycogen. Glycogen is the body's main substance for sugar and is stored in the liver as glucose for later use by the adrenals.

Diabetes occurs due to deficient action in insulin and hypoglycemia due to excess action.

Glucagon Hormone

Opposite to therole of insulin, glucagon's function is to re-convert glycogen stored in the cells and liver into sugar. It is then returned to the bloodstream as an available source of energy, with the purpose of preventing blood sugar levels from getting too low. Another function is to precipitate the break down and stimulate and conversion of protein into sugars. This function is also shared with the adrenal cortex hormones and the pituitary growth hormone.

Glucagon also plays an important role in maintaining a salt

and fluid balance in our bodies. When we are depleted of sugar and salt due to excessive sweating, from over-exertion for example, glucagon kicks in to re-establish balance. Hypoglycemia is a result of a deficiency or excess in glucagon. Foods that naturally contain magnesium, potassium, or sodium will help to stimulate the correct functioning of this gland.

Symptom Repertory:

Physiological	Emotional/Mental
Abnormal blood cholesterol	Constant anxiety
Continual thirst	Memory lapses
Dehydration	Mood swings
Excessive appetite	Teary
Excessive urination	
Fatigue	
Heavy smoking	
Increased abdominal fat	
Low/high blood sugar	
Nervous disturbances of the stomach	
Poor circulation to extremities	
Salt imbalances	
Skin changes	
Sugar cravings	

Natural Corrective Measures

- Manage your weight levels.

- Monitor sugar and alcohol intake.

- Foods loaded with vitamin C, carotenoids, folate and

fibersuch as dark leafy greens like spinach, kale, brassica family such as broccoli and brussel sprouts, orange-yellow vegetables such as squash, sweet potatoes, and carrots.

- Avoid prepared or processed foods.

- Foods that naturally contain magnesium, potassium or sodium will help to stimulate the correct functioning of this gland.

NB refer to Part Three — Putting it All Together — *Herbs and Foods for Healthy Endocrine.*

Adrenals

["The Adrenals ... its primary function is to regulate the four primary stress hormones: DHEA, adrenaline, cortisol and norepinephrine"]

Known as the *glands of combat* because they respond swiftly to rage, anger, and fear, the adrenal glands are the survival center of the human body — the seat of the flight or fight responses.

Situated at the top of both kidneys, the adrenals are triangular and orange-colored the size of Brazil nuts. They regulate adrenalin and react strongly to unhealthy mental and emotional conditions.

Traditional Chinese medicine and the western visionary Edgar Cayce both say the adrenals are the storehouse of one's emotional karma in the body.

The adrenals stimulate sexual expression, so when in a hypoactive state due to exhaustion of the sympathetic responses or high toxicity, the sex glands weaken diminishing sex drive.

Each gland consists of a medulla (the center of the gland) and the adrenal cortex.

Adrenal Medulla

The Adrenal Medulla produces two hormones adrenalin and nor-adrenalin and create a variety of effects in the body, most of which can be regarded as preparing it for flight or fight. In the event of enormous stress, glycogen which is stored in the liver is released as sugar/glucose to the adrenals for extra energy.

Both of these hormones are often linked with psychiatric disorders involving depression and elation - manic depressives. Medical sources say that the degree of aggression in a personality is related to the relative proportion of adrenalin of nor-adrenalin. For example, an aggressive person has relatively less nor-adrenalin. Adrenalin is the rush and nor-adrenalin is the lull.

Adrenalin is also invaluable in the process of releasing toxins from the body. It produces other hormones necessary for fluid and electrolyte (salt) balance in the body such as cortisone and aldosterone.

Adrenal Cortex

The adrenal cortex is largely dependent upon adrenocorti-cotrotropic hormone or ACTH released by the pituitary gland. A deficiency in this important hormone leads to fluctuations in blood pressure levels, and in particular a tendency towards low blood pressure. It can also result in a craving for carbohydrates or salt and to decreased metabolism. Where there is a deficiency in this hormone an inability to metabolize carbohydrates and a drop in the production of insulin by the pancreas often follows, leading to high levels of blood sugar and the condition known as diabetes.

The adrenal cortex influences the development and mainte-nance of secondary sex characteristics and increases the deposition of protein in muscles and the reduction of nitrogen in males. When there is hyper-secretion of the hormones in adults, females develop male attributes and vice versa.

The adrenal cortex hormones are crucial in helping one to adapt to all sorts of stresses, trauma and disease as it releases anti-stress hormones that relax the muscles and resort harmony. They also affect the control of mood and blood pressure, and very importantly the metabolic reactions involving carbohydrates and protein food stuffs. It also includes the re-absorption of sodium via the kidneys and the elimination of potassium.

Adrenal Over-load

Because of the many stressful situations encountered everyday, the adrenal secretions are subject to depletion or weakening. In a stressed state, our body increases its production of stress hormones (cortisol, cortisone, and adrenaline) to allow us to cope with stress better. In a normal situation, the adrenals defuse stress and restores balance.

But if the adrenals are compromised or weakened, the release of stress hormones serves to set up a situation where the body is bombarded with 'stress hormones'. When this occurs, white blood cell production and function is inhibited, particularly the production of natural killer cells which ward off infection. Rather than being able to release the stress and allow for a natural state of relaxation, the body is pushed into 'stress mode' — this is the condition of adrenal overload.

How does a weakening occur?

Adrenal over-load can occur due to a number of lifestyle factors such as:

- Over-use of stimulants such as caffeine. In the short term the coffee gives more energy, however, over time, the continued stimulation drains the adrenals leading to fatigue, low back pain, sleeping disorders, hyper-vigilant states, anxiety and leaching of nutrients from the body

- Sugar and other refined carbohydrates are other culprits, and the stimulation from these on the adrenals depletes B vitamins from the body

- Emotional stress

- Poor sleeping habits

- Overwork or exertion

- Hyper-vigilant states such as anxiety and panic attacks

- Pharmaceutical drugs

- Many of these are the cause of adrenal overload and a symptom of, as they generate a perpetuated cycle which can result in a final burn-out.

Adrenal over-load is a condition created by pro-longed stress. When stressed or in drain mode, the adrenals panic, and this forces the kidneys to go into spasm which creates the urge to pass water. Sustained states of panic means that nutrients do not get the opportunity to be assimilated by the body with the increased need to pass water. This can lead to dehydration, inability to assimilate and absorb nutrients and vital minerals and vitamins. This creates long term pressure on the adrenals as they are in a constant state of output or panic.

The symptoms of adrenal exhaustion are varied and occur over a prolonged period of time during which one endures enormous stress such as living in an unhappy relationship, working excessively long hours or strenuous pressure on the body due to physical labor or over-exercising.

Symptom Repertory: (Adrenal Exhaustion)

Physiological	Emotional/Mental
Aggressive behavior or outbursts	Constant weariness
Allergies/Asthma	Depression
Arthritis	Easily irritated
Bone loss	Fears
Bruising easily	Highs and lows in moods and behaviours
Caffeine cravings	Hypertension
Chemical sensitivities	Inability to cope with stress
Dark circle under the eyes	Memory lapses
Dehydration	Mood swings
Endocrine imbalances	Phobias

Excessive thirst

Hair loss

High blood pressure

High blood sugar

Inability to metabolize
carbohydrates

Increased need to pass
urine

Increased sensitivity to
odor (both pleasant
and unpleasant)

Low back pain

Low blood pressure

Potassium deficiency

Salt craving

Sleep disorders

Sugar cravings

Panic Attacks

Schizophrenia

A Self-test to Check Adrenal Health:

You will need a blood pressure monitor.

1. Lie down and rest for five minutes.

2. After five minutes, take your blood pressure (while lying down).

3. Next, stand up and immediately take another reading.

If your blood pressure is lower after you stand up, your adrenals may be functioning poorly.

[Note: this test is designed for self-care management, it is not designed to take the role of your professional health practitioner.]

Natural Corrective Measures

- Maintain acid/alkaline balance within the body

- Stress management techniques such relaxation

- Twenty minutes of meditation daily

- Yoga

- Drink plenty of water to flush kidneys

- Laughter has an anti-stress effect on the body. It can lower serum cortisol and adrenaline. Smile and laugh more often.

NB refer to Part Three: Putting it All Together — *Herbs and Foods for Healthy Endocrine.*

Gonads

["The Gonads ... primary function is the creation of the sex hormones"]

The primary function of the gonads is the creation of the sex hormones and they also govern the development of secondary sexual characteristics and sexual activity.

Ovaries

The ovaries are a pair of female reproductive organs located in the pelvis, one on each side of the uterus. They are connected to each other by the fallopian tubes and are part of a woman's reproductive system.

The ovaries produce eggs in the ovaries and influence female characteristics. They also produce three hormones:

- Progesterone
- Estrogen
- Testosterone

Estrogen

Estrogen is a group of female sex hormones that stimulate the appearance of secondary female sex characteristics in girls at puberty. Estrogen controls the growth of the lining of the uterus during the first part of the menstrual cycle, creates breast development in pregnancy and regulates various metabolic processes.

Estrogen has a number of physiological effects:

- Restrains bone loss
- Creates progesterone receptors
- Reduces vascular tone (dilates blood vessels)

- Creates proliferative endometrium
- Salt and fluid retention
- Relieves hot flashes
- Prevents vaginal dryness & mucosal atrophy
- Improves memory
- Improves sleep disorders
- Improves health of urinary tract
- Relieves night sweats

Progesterone

Progesterone is made in the ovaries of menstruating women and by the placenta during pregnancy. It is naturally secreted by the ovary in the second two weeks of the menstrual cycle in reproductive age ovulating women.

Progesterone has a number of physiological effects, often regulatory:

- Protects against breast fibro cysts
- Helps use fat for energy
- Natural diuretic
- Natural anti-depressant & calms anxiety
- Prevents cyclical migraines
- Promotes normal sleep patterns
- Facilitates thyroid hormone function
- Helps normalize blood sugar levels
- Normalizes blood clotting
- Helps restores normal libido
- Normalizes zinc and copper levels
- Restores proper cell oxygen levels
- Prevents endometrial cancer and helps prevent breast cancer
- Stimulates new bone formation
- Improves vascular tone
- Prevents autoimmune diseases

Testosterone

Testosterone is known as the male hormone, but women produce small amounts throughout their lives — about one-seventh the amount per day that men make.

In women, testosterone is produced half in the ovaries and half in the adrenal glands. After menopause, testosterone production decreases gradually by one third of pre-menopausal levels (unlike estrogen production which decreases dramatically). Testosterone levels drop by half if the ovaries are removed.

Testosterone in women helps maintain muscle and bone mass and contributes to the libido.

Symptom Repertory Female Hormone Deficiency:

Estrogen Deficiency	Testosterone Deficiency	Progesterone Deficiency
Bloating	Aches/pains	See Table below,
Constant fatigue	Depressed	Estrogen excess
Depression	Fatigue	forces a deficiency
Dry skin	Foggy Head	in Progesterone.
Headaches	Incontinence	
Hot flashes	Low libido	
Impaired memory	Memory lapses	
Joint pain, swelling	Sleep disorders	
and stiffness	Vaginal dryness	
Loss of libido		
Low Back Pain		
Night sweats		
Osteoarthritis		
Memory lapses		
Rapid pulse rate		
Sleep disorders		

Unexplained
   weight gain
Urinary tract
   infections

Symptom Repertory Female Hormone Excess:

Estrogen dominance/ Too little progesterone	Progesterone Excess	Testosterone Excess
Allergies	Acne	Excessive facial/ body hair
Autoimmune	Breast swelling	Increased acne
Bloating	Depression	Oliy skin
Blood clotting	Digestive	Head hair loss
Blood sugar	problems	Decreased HDL
imbalance	Dizziness	(good cholesterol)
Breast tenderness	Euphoria	
Chronic fatigue	Sleepiness	
syndrome	Yeast Infection	
Cold hands and		
feet		
Copper retention		
Cyclical migraines		
Depression		
Dry eyes		
Endometriosis		
Fatigue		
Foggy head		
Gallbladder disease		
Hair loss		
Headaches		
Incontinence		

Increased body fat
Infertility
Insomnia
Irritability
Little or no libido
Magnesium
    deficiency
Memory loss
Menstrual problems
Miscarriages/
    infertility
Mood swings
Osteoporosis
PMS
Premenopausal
    bone loss
Premature aging
Sluggish metabolism
Uterine fibroids
Yeast infections
Zinc, loss of

Testes

The testes are male glands which secrete testosterone, which stimulates sperm production and development of male characteristics.

Testosterone is a steroid hormone derived from cholesterol. It is the principal male sex hormone and an anabolic steroid. In both males and females, it plays a key role in health and wellbeing. Examples include enhanced libido, energy, immune function, and protection against osteoporosis. On average, the adult male body produces about twenty times the amount of testosterone that an adult female's body does·

Testosterone is responsible for the following changes in males:

- Increased libido and erection frequency
- Facial hair (sideburns, beard, moustache)
- Subcutaneous fat in face decreases
- Increased muscle strength and mass
- Deepening of voice
- Growth of the Adam's apple
- Growth of spermatogenesis tissue in testes, male fertility
- Growth of jaw, brow, chin, nose
- Shoulders widen and rib cage expands
- Completion of bone maturation and termination of growth.

Symptom Repertory:

Physiological	Emotional/Mental
Bone loss	Decreased stamina
Decreased muscle strength	Decreased mental clarity
Decreased urine flow	Depression
Erectile dysfunction	Irritability
Hot flashes	Mood swings

Increased abdominal fat
Increased urge to urinate
Loss of libido
Night sweats
Poor concentration
Sleep disorders

Natural Corrective Measures

- Increase natural hormones found in herbs and plants
- Yoga

NB refer to Part Three: Putting it All Together — *Herbs and Foods for Healthy Endocrine*

Holistic Relationships —
the Endocrine System and the:

- **Immune System**
- **Reproductive System**
- **Nervous System**
- **Circulatory System**
- **Respiratory System**
- **Digestive System**
- **Skeletal System**
- **Excretory/Urinary System**
- **Muscular System**

Holistic Relationships — Interactions with Other Systems

The endocrine system is a part of many other systems within the body. Each system has its own unique patterns and processes in addition to working with each other towards a homeostatic state.

We can assist the role of the endocrine system through an understanding of these systems and their relationship with these systems.

Eight Systems of the Human Body

1. Endocrine system — *flow of hormones*
2. Immune system — *flow of defense*
3. Reproductive System — *flow of life*
4. Nervous system — *flow of communication*
5. Circulatory system — *flow of blood*
6. Respiratory system — *flow of air*
7. Digestive system — *flow nutrition*
8. Skeletal system — *flow of structure protection framework*
9. Excretory/Urinary system — *flow of elimination*
10. Muscular system — *flow of movement*

The Immune System

["The Immune System — flow of defense"]

Purpose

The immune system is one of the most complex and amazing systems in the human body. Its primary role is to protect the body against infection and prevent the development of disease and cancer. Simply, the purpose of the immune system is to defend. It is our first line of defense against disease and infection such as viruses, fungi and bacteria as well as cancer.

The system is comprised of a network of immune cells and antibodies, which circulate through the blood, lymphatic vessels and organs such as lymph nodes, thymus, spleen, adenoids, appendix and tonsils, they fight against microbes.

When our immune system is under-functioning we are prone to disease, infection, allergies, hypersensitivities and immune system disorders.

Endocrine System and the Immune System

The endocrine system plays an important role with the immune system. They work collaboratively at many levels defending the body and supporting overall health.

The thymus gland is the major gland of the immune system. It is a prime site for the production of white blood cells and helps to make T lymphocytes and issues commands to these cells regarding which enemies to attack. It also plays an integral role in the flow of lymph throughout the body.

The spleen filters foreign invaders out from the blood. It is responsible for producing white blood cells, engulfing and destroying bacteria and cellular debris, destroying worn-out red blood cells and platelets, coordinating the interaction between macrophages, antibodies, T lymphocytes and B-Lymphocytes and acting as a blood reservoir. The spleen also releases many potent immune-system-enhancing compounds.

The adrenals provide the fight or flight reactors when the body comes under attack from infection.

The pituitary releases the growth hormone which stimulates the immune system.

The pineal releases melatonin which is useful in fighting infectious disease including viral infections.

The Immune System and relationship glands:

- Spleen
- Thymus
- Adrenals
- Pituitary
- Pineal

The Nervous System

["The nervous system — flow of communication"]

Purpose
In a nutshell, the main purpose of the nervous system is about communication. That is — sending, receiving and processing nerve impulses throughout the body. The main organs in the nervous system are the brain, spinal cord and nerves.

Without the nervous system our body would fail to operate at an alarming rate, messages would become skewiff and as a result, the body would begin to break down.

Endocrine System and the Nervous System
The endocrine system and the nervous system work together in harmony and communication of the internal environment to maintain homeostasis. The brain receives input from the outer and inner environments, and sends messages to the body via the pituitary and the pineal. These messages are passed down through the body to other glands.

The adrenals react to mental and emotional stresses by secreting hormones which excite the body to fight or flee, continued excitement or stress will exhaust the body.

The hormones released by the thyroid influence nerve stability and proper nerve activity.

The Nervous System and relationship to glands:

- Adrenals
- Thyroid
- Pituitary
- Pineal

The Circulatory System

["The Circulatory System — flow of blood"]

Purpose

The major components of the circulatory system are the heart, arteries, blood vessels, lymphatic and veins. The main purpose of this system is to circulate blood and oxygen throughout the body. The heart pumps blood to the arteries. The arteries take the oxygenated blood to the muscles. The veins take blood back to the heart, which then releases carbon dioxide in the lungs.

Endocrine System and the Circulatory System

Each gland of the endocrine system has its arterial and venous blood supply. Lack of oxygen in the blood stream has a direct affect upon the adrenal medulla and adrenal hormones.

In the event of 'flight or fight' stress, the release of adrenal hormones, adrenaline and nor-adrenaline, influence dilatory stimulations which increases blood supply, oxygen supply and blood pressure. Blood pressure is also raised by the anti-diuretic hormone of the pituitary posterior lobe when the blood vessels are contracted.

The endocrine system secretes hormones into the blood stream for circulation to parts of the body necessary for processes such as metabolism, growth, inner stability, resistance to stress and reproductive cycles. Poor circulation means that hormones take longer to reach their destination and this influences these vital processes.

The Circulatory System and relationship glands:

- Adrenals
- Pituitary
- Thyroid

The Respiratory System

["The Respiratory System — flow of air"]

Purpose

The respiratory system is more than the process of breathing in and out. Its purpose is more complex than that, although breathing in and out is a way in which this system operates. Essentially, the respiratory system brings oxygen into the blood so it can distribute it to the cells of the body.

That familiar mantra — "breathe in the good and breathe out the bad —" is more than a mantra or over-used new age cliché. Breathing is a mechanism of cleansing, nourishment, rejuvenation and restoration. It is a miraculous system of balance, bringing about a state of homeostasis.

Breathing — cleanses. As we breathe out, the respiratory system takes the carbon dioxide out of the blood.

Breathing — nourishes. As we breathe in, oxygen transmutes into nutrients.

Breathing — rejuvenates. As we breathe in, we take air into the lungs and this puts oxygen into the blood rejuvenating our cells. As we breathe out, stale air is expelled thus assisting the rejuvenation process.

Breathing — restores. The processes of the respiratory system helps to regulate the body's pH acid/alkaline balance.

Breathing — balances and brings about a state of homeostasis. When we remember to breathe. Yet often times we forget to breathe, and when we do, we halt or interrupt these important processes. Why do we forget to breathe? Naturally, it isn't a conscious moment, but we forget to breathe when we over-think, in moments of fear, grief, anger, sorrow or failing to be present moment and fully aware.

However, if we use breath to breathe through and into our emotions such as fear, grief, sorrow or anger, we harmonize the emotion which brings about balance to the respiratory system and diffuses the emotion allowing them to dissipate through the out-breath. The same principle applies to over-thinking. Bringing awareness to the breath re-focuses our thoughts and we re-establish control, that is — we control the thought, breathe and the thoughts move on and out through the breath.

The major organs in the respiratory system are the lungs, trachea, bronchioles, mouth, nose and epiglottis.

Endocrine System and the Respiratory System
Movement of air through the throat affects the thyroid and parathyroid gland processes. For example, in the event of stress or shallow breathing, the throat constricts inhibiting air flow. Conversely, the thyroid gland affects the respiratory processes as the thyroxine and triiodothyronine hormones increases oxygen consumption.

In addition, the adrenal medulla affects respiratory function as it secretes in response to sympathetic stimulation and causes dilation of the bronchi allowing a higher intake of air per breath.

The Respiratory System and relationship glands:

- Thyroid
- Parathyroid
- Adrenal Medulla

The Digestive System

["The Digestive System — flow of nutrition"]

Purpose

The digestive system includes the mouth, esophagus, liver, stomach, large intestine and small intestine. The purpose of this system is not just about digesting food. It starts with the process of salivation, which gets the digestive juices running. Once food is taken into the mouth, it is chewed. The food goes down the esophagus, then into the stomach where it combines with hydrochloric acid in the stomach. This then passes into the small intestines and then into the large intestine. The rest is left up to the excretory system.

Endocrine System and the Digestive System

The endocrine system plays its role primarily through the thyroid gland as it governs the basic metabolism of digestion. Thyroid activity influences the rate that digestion moves through the bowels, thus affecting the absorption of nutrients. Thyroid hormones - thyroxine and triiodothyronine — influence carbohydrate absorption and metabolism. Hyper-thyroidism causes loss of weight together with increase of appetite.

Additionally, the adrenals affect the digestive system through the nervous system. Adrenal stimulation limits saliva flow so that energy is released for 'flight or fight'.

Secretions of the adrenal cortex regulate the carbohydrate metabolism, the change of glycogen to glucose, and the utilization of carbohydrates derived from proteins.

Pituitary secretions of the anterior lobe affect protein anabolism, absorption of calcium for the bowel and conversion of glycogen to glucose, all related to growth activity.

The pancreas plays a vital role in digestion through secretions to the liver where it breaks down sugar to store or increase sugar concentration in the blood. This also affects the breakdown and metabolism of fatty acids and the conversion of amino acids to glucose. Beta cells secrete the protein insulin and influence uptake of sugar.

The Digestive System and relationship glands:

- Thyroid
- Pituitary
- Adrenals
- Pancreas

The Skeletal System

["The Skeletal System — flow of structure protection framework"]

Purpose
The skeletal system has a purpose; it gives the human body shape and support. It protects other parts of our body, like the brain, lungs, heart and liver, allowing bodily movement, producing blood cells, and storing minerals. This system consists of 206 different size and shaped bones, cartilage, and joints.

Endocrine System and the Skeletal System
The anterior lobe of the pituitary secretes growth hormones which determine bone structure and absorption of calcium from the bowel.

The relationship of the para-thyroids and the skeletal is important to the skeletal system and to the calcium production in the blood.

The Skeletal System and relationship glands:

- Pituitary
- Parathyroid
- Thyroid

The Excretory/Urinary System

["The Excretory/Urinary System — flow of elimination"]

Purpose

The excretory system connects to the digestive system. Its purpose is to eliminate waste and toxins from the body. Additionally, this system helps to regulate blood pressure, metabolism, and blood composition and volume. The main organs of the excretory system are the bladder, ureters, urethra, kidneys, lungs, liver and skin.

Endocrine System and the Excretory System

The pituitary gland posterior lobe secretes anti-diuretic hormone which maintains the body's water balance and adjusts osmotic pressure.

The hypothalamus stimulates or inhibits this secretion and lack of this hormone results in over excretion of urine. This is also the case when the adrenals are over-stimulated. Conversely, sympathetic stimulation of the adrenal gland inhibits bladder function.

The adrenal cortex is involved with water metabolism and controls excretion of potassium and re-absorption of sodium, when adrenal hormones are inadequate the kidneys excrete too much sodium and this can cause Addison's disease.

The Excretory/Urinary System and relationship glands:

- Pituitary
- Hypothalamus
- Adrenal

The Muscular System

["The Muscular System — flow of movement"]

Purpose
The human body contains more than 650 individual muscles, which are attached to the skeleton. Working in harmony with the skeletal system its primary purpose is to provide the pulling power for us to move around.

The Muscular System includes three types of muscles:

- *smooth,* found on the walls of internal organs
- *cardiac,* found only in the heart
- *skeletal* muscles, which help strengthen the body and connect to bones

Endocrine System and the Muscular System
The thyroid hormones generate growth of skin and hair which support the muscular system. The parathyroid hormones influence support the production of calcium.

The growth hormone secreted by the pituitary play an important role in the development of the muscular system. For example, the anti-diuretic hormone released by the pituitary posterior lobe contracts the *smooth* muscles of the internal organs. Skin pigmentation is affected by the secretions of the middle lobe of the pituitary.

Over (hyper) stimulation of the adrenals can create 'goose flesh' and increased sweat glands. Hyper-secretions from the adrenal cortex, creates muscle wasting due to protein breakdown excesses, and muscular weakness due to potassium loss through kidneys takes place.

The Muscular System and relationship glands:

- Thyroid
- Parathyroid
- Pituitary
- Adrenal

PART TWO: THE SUBTLE BODY

Symptoms of Health

Health in a human being,
is the perfection of bodily organization,
intellectual energy,
and moral power.
Health is,
the fullest expression of all the faculties and passions of man,
acting together in perfect harmony.
Health is,
entire freedom from pain of body and
discordance of mind.
Health is,
beauty, energy,
purity, holiness,
happiness.
Health is,
that condition in which,
man is the highest known expression of power and
goodness of his Maker.
When a man is perfect in his own nature,
body and soul,
perfect in their harmonious adoptions and action,
and living in perfect harmony with nature,
with his fellow man,
and with his God,
he may be said to be in a state of health.

~ Dr Nichols "Our Medical Books" 1853 ~

Metaphysical Processes

["Health is a state of complete harmony of the body, mind and spirit. When one is free from physical disabilities and mental distractions, the gates of the soul open."]

~ B.K.S. Iyengar ~

- **The Subtle Body Systems**
- **The Aura**
- **The Nadis**
- **The Meridians**
- **The Chakras**

Metaphysical, a word steeped in mystery and often misunderstood. As a derivative of the word *metaphysics*, metaphysical relates to the science of *that which transcends the physical*.

To gain a deeper understanding (and maybe allay misunderstanding) *metaphysical* is a combination of *meta* from the Greek — 'in the midst of, in common with, in pursuit or quest of' and *physical* from M.L. — 'of nature, study of nature.'

It was much later that it was characterized by the meaning of 'bodily attributes or activities.'

And so, metaphysical means — in common with or in pursuit or quest of the physical nature. And so … we begin the next part of the journey — the metaphysical processes.

["… we are more than just our physical bodies …"]

We have discussed the physiological processes of the human body in relation to the endocrine system. In this chapter we discuss the metaphysical processes of the human body in relation to the endocrine system.

The subject of metaphysics and associated processes is

integral to the practice of holism towards achieving sustainable health. It is a subject that has been around for centuries.

Ancient physicians attributed great importance to the emotions and the mind in the healing processes, often times more so than physical aches and pains. This supports the theory of holism or totalism, and pays precedence to the notion that we inherently possess great powers of healing. Today, this is an acceptable and sort-after notion and if applied, one can enhance the processes of sustainable health.

As a system, it addresses the human being in its entirety, the principle being that each of aspects of our being — emotional, mental and physical — work in a cooperative manner, integrated and in harmony towards optimal wellbeing engendering a state of homeostasis.

In the same vein, holistic practice encompasses many modalities including the collaboration of both conventional medicines with alternative practices. For example, an individual could be receiving treatment for a physiological condition such as an injury, through a trusted conventional practice and couple this treatment with an alternative practice such as acupuncture. Or one could be using conventional practices to heal an illness whilst supporting the emotional and mental aspects through counseling, yoga or massage.

And so it is, integral to the holism theory is the understanding that we are more than just our physical bodies. We are beings of mind, body and soul/spirit. Our being, in its totality or entirety, is dependant upon the interaction between the physical body and the subtle body.

To Summarize ...

Our personal tuning fork or physiological system is not complete without its counter-part, the subtle energies.

An understanding of our physiological-being is enhanced through an understanding of our subtle energies via an understanding of metaphysics, encompassing:

Physiological — the study of the physical body and its processes vital to optimum health and wellbeing.

Metaphysics or Metaphysical — the understanding or study which deals with the first causes of things.

Subtle Body — the study of the metaphysical body and its processes vital to optimum health and wellbeing.

~

- Our true state of health is not a goal to be reached merely by the study of the physiological processes but as a cooperative collaboration of the physiological, metaphysical and subtle body processes.

- True health requires a balanced and fluid connection between the physical body and the subtle body in order to maintain this dynamic state.

- Then, health will not be merely a goal to be reached but rather, a dynamic place of wellbeing.

The Subtle Body Systems

- **Pathways of Energy**
- **The Flow of Life**
- **The Systems**

The word subtle is from Old French *soutil*, from Latin *subtilis* 'fine, thin, delicate, finely woven.' From sub — 'under' + -tilis — 'web.'

And so … our subtle body — as part of the metaphysical system — is a delicate and finely woven matrix of pathways which interact with the physical body with every breath we take. Moreover, esoteric teachings demonstrate this interaction occurs with every lifetime, every thought pattern and every level of consciousness.

The subtle bodies are our individual pathways representing life-support systems. As keys to blocked and stored energy they are essential to a balanced and harmonious existence.

Pathways of Energy

Einstein's discovery that the universe is a collection of atoms helps us to understand the human body as an energetic system. If we broke down our body into small units we would find it composed of millions of cells. Break these down further and we find subatomic particles. All of which vibrate as patterns of energy.

These patterns of energy have their own unique blueprint and molecular structure in terms of our DNA. To function — that is to provide life to the physical form — these patterns require flow and to flow.

The Flow of Life

["This energetic system influences and gives life to the physical body."]

The physical body is constituted by dense systems and a mass physical form thus the subtle body, by virtue of this solidity, is subtler. So too are the systems that the subtle body houses. These systems are energetic by nature and it is here that we find the link to the physical body in the endocrine system.

Whilst the endocrine system is part of the physical body, when it is in a state of calibration it operates at a finely tuned level delivering vital messages between the subtle and physical bodies. The endocrine system therefore, has the ability to enable a state of homeostasis towards sustainable health for our system as a whole.

As an operating system integral to sustainable health, the endocrine system performs this function via an output and input flow of breath or chi — an ever present, ever flowing exchange of energy. It occurs as a participation of processes between the physical and subtle body.

The flow is smooth and operational:

Physical Body—Endocrine System—Subtle Body—Subtle Body—Endocrine System—Physical Body

The flow influences, permeates and gives life: An interruption of this flow creates an imbalance of energies at either a physical or subtle body level — homeostasis is interrupted — sustainable health is inhibited. An interruption can occur at any level, in any system or through any stage of our holistic process.

The Systems

["... subtle systems serve their own purpose towards higher evolvement, health, emotions ..."]

In much the same way that the Physical Body houses many systems, the Subtle Body houses many systems. These systems possess their own modus operandi — each with its own corresponding vehicle of consciousness beyond all of which is the spiritual-soul principle.

Thus each of these subtle systems serve their own purpose towards higher evolvement, in terms of health, emotions, spiritual development and mental consciousness.

The Subtle Body systems comprise of:

- **Aura** — the energetic emanation surrounding the physical form

- **Nadis** — three channels distributing pranic/chi energy to the chakras

- **Meridians** — 14 energy pathways distributing pranic/chi energy to the endocrine system and physical body

- **Chakras** — energetic vortices located along the major meridians

As you journey through this system of energies — a developed understanding will occur of how the aura, chakras and meridians act as essential aspects of holistic therapy practice. Essentially, they contribute as a gateway to good health and wellbeing.

A balanced energy system with a clean and clear aura, balanced chakras and flowing meridians free of energy blockages will reflect in good health, balanced moods and emotions, mental agility and reduced stress and a comfortable and contented spiritual outlook.

~

Thus homeostasis is achieved ... and the journey goes on ... in health ... sustainable and with all systems working together as a *totalism*.

The Aura

["Aura — the energetic emanation surrounding the physical form."]

- **Light Waves in Motion**
- **Layers, Planes and Sheaths**
- **The Hierarchy of Disease**
- **Exercises to Sense, See, Feel the Aura**
- **Balancing, Cleansing the Aura**
- **The Characteristics of the Aura**
- **The Seven Layers of the Aura**

Aura — originating from Greek meaning *breath* or *breeze*. In 1859 a newer translation occurred — *subtle emanation around living beings*. In metaphysics, the human aura is the same — an energy field emanating from the surface of a person or objects and can be seen as swirling vibrations of color.

Light Waves in Motion

["... the human body emanates energy, a universal energy field — the aura."]

The auric phenomenon has been observed for centuries. Perceived as a luminous body it was first recorded in western literature by the Pythagoreans around 500BC. They held that its light could produce a variety of effects in the human organism, including curing illness. Einstein spoke about our aura as light waves in motion. He was one of the first scientists to develop a theory re the connection between matter and energy. His theory is vital in understanding the human form as more than a physical mass. Indeed, his work demonstrated, we emanate energy — and if the human body emanates energy, then there must be a universal energy field — the aura.

Einstein's work spurred research by Dr William Kilner of St. Thomas Hospital in 1910. Kilner grasped the theory that all matter consists of energy and saw a correlation between this energy and the aura. He designed a special screen called a Kilner screen which comprised of a set of lenses coated with dicyanin dye. From here he conducted a series of investigations where he observed a glowing mist around the body in the form of three zones. Kilner found that this aura differed considerably according to age, gender, mental and emotional states, and health. Certain disease presented as patches, discoloration or irregularities. He went on to diagnose on this basis. Unfortunately, Kilner met with substantial ridicule and resistance from fellow medical professionals. Like other pioneers in medical history he revolutionized the way we think about health and our form as a human being but at a cost.

Kilner's work was not unfounded and in the 1920s French Physicist Louis De Broglie developed the concept of matter waves. His research postulated that every particle of matter can be replaced by an energy wave which constitutes as the aura. In essence, De Broglie's work supported the theory that the human body is more than a solid mass; indeed it has an energy field. Unlike Kilner's work, De Broglie's work received some theoretical recognition culminating in a Nobel Prize in 1923.

With still much to be proven re the existence of the human aura at a scientific level, in the 1950's Professor Harold Saxton Burr successfully measured the electrical nature of the human form. He too, found that this energetic field varied in emanation according to states of health and in particular emotional states. This was a revolutionary breakthrough in terms of holistic health.

Burr's work met with similar disdain as did Kilner's, however in the 1960s Russian scientists repeated his work and verified that indeed it is a momentous concept and reason why the aura existed — that is to provide a pathway for healing.

Layers, Planes and Sheaths

["... shifting, pulsating ... it breathes life force energy into the physical form."]

The aura comprises difference layers. Most teachings discuss seven as the primary layers, each layer becoming thinner or finer the further from the human physical form. These seven layers act as a multi-layered shell of energy which interacts with the energies of our environment. Always shifting, pulsating and vibrating, it breathes life force energy into the physical form.

~ Ketheric
~ Celestial
~ Causal
~ Astral
~ Mental
~ Emotional
~ Etheric

In much the same way, the Earth can be viewed as having a similar emanation ... or aura. Earth's energetic emanations are evidenced in the atmospheric layers and are analogous to the layers of the human aura.

For example:

~ The Troposphere
~ The Stratosphere
~ The Mesosphere
~ The Thermosphere
~ The Exosphere
~ The Ionosphere
~ The Magnetosphere

These layers are never still always pulsating and shifting — there is a constant exchange of energy — an input and output between the physical form and layers or planes of consciousness.

Each of these seven layers comprise individual and interrelated planes of consciousness:

~ The spiritual plane
~ The astral plane
~ The physical plane

• The **spiritual plane** is our direct link with the spirit consciousness. It has the highest vibration of the auric planes and metabolizes energy related to the spiritual world. This is the world of our invisible sensations and experiences.

Aura layers associated with the **spiritual plane**:

~ Ketheric Layer
~ Celestial Layer
~ Causal Layer

• The **astral plane** is the connecting plane between the physical and spiritual. It is the blueprint to our spiritual potential. Associated with unconditional love it is the doorway through which we can energy into the other states of reality. Spiritual energy passes through here to be transformed into physical energy and vice versa.

Aura layers associated with the **astral plane**:

~ Astral Layer

• The **physical plane** is responsible for the transfer of life energy or vitality from the universal energy field to the physical body and metabolizes energies related to the physical world. This is the world of our five senses and all physical sensations.

Aura layers associated with the **physical plane**:

~ Mental Layer
~ Emotional Layer
~ Etheric Layer
~ Physical Body

As an emanation of energy the aura acts as a container and a conduit exchanging information with the universe according to the layers and their associated planes of consciousness. As a principle of nature it keeps humans evolving through spirit whilst remaining in physical existence.

The Hierarchy of Disease

[*"... healing is dependant upon a holistic approach, encompassing the aura, chakras and physical body."*]

As a 3-dimensional multi-layered shell of pulsating energies, the aura is usually about 22 times larger than the human form. However it can vary in size according to feelings and state of health. For example when we greet a friend we are happy to see, our aura can expand emanating warmth. Conversely, when in a situation of fear or feeling grief or sorrow our aura can contract, appear cool and sometimes sharper. Furthermore, the structure of the human aura grows and changes according to spiritual and physical growth patterns. It is likened to that of a record-holder of all lives experiences.

There has been much discussion in relation to the aura and

disease. In particular the notion the physical body is the last point of manifestation in terms of disease. This notion explores the journey of disease in terms of a system of hierarchy and begins in the aura first as a blockage in one of the sheaths or layers which shifts to the chakras which is then distributed to the endocrine system and finally manifests in the physical body via its other systems.

Following this hierarchy, healing is dependant upon a holistic approach, encompassing the aura, chakras and physical body.

When the aura is supported and strengthened it has the ability to act as a protective zone between the physical body and the outside world. In much the same way a house provides shelter and protection from the elements. It works in harmony with the chakras to vitalize the physical body which feeds the meridians and then on to the endocrine system and the other systems of the body. In this way, the endocrine system acts as a conduit between the subtle body and physical body.

Exercises to Sense, See, Feel the Aura

Seeing the Aura

Some people possess a natural ability to see or sense auras. Learning to see auras is not as difficult as one may think and it does require a willingness to open the mind to the concept.

1. First thing first, relax and decide that you are open to this experience.

2. Find a mirror that is in a well lit room.

3. Breathe in and out gently, and focus on your head and shoulder area.

4. Remain still, and in the gently breathing state, attempt to

keep your focus on this area.

5. Soon you should be able to see the electromagnetic energies as a field of light, circling around your head.

This same process can be conducted on a plant or tree or another person. With practice you may be able to see colors, shapes or dark spots which could indicate a weakness in the auric field.

Sensing the Aura

Exercise one
Perhaps you feel more attuned to the process of sensing auras. Many times we intuitively sense another's aura and can manifest as an overall feeling of comfort or discomfort, coolness or warmth, or tingly sensations. Discomfort may generate as feeling tired, drained or uneasy. Conversely you could feel relaxed, uplifted or experience a feeling of having known this person before.

As a more mechanical exercise to sense the aura and its electromagnetic energies:

1. Close your eyes and rub the palms of the hands together to generate warmth.

2. Hold the palms of your hand facing each other about two inches apart.

3. Slowly move the hands out and back in.

4. Pushing the hands out further with each movement.

5. After a few seconds you should begin to feel a ball of energy between the hands.

6. Once you are confident in sensing the energy, open your eyes to see the energy. Positioning yourself towards natural light will help this.

7. Try moving your palms further and further apart slowly. See how far you can go before you no longer feel the pull.

8. Now try pointing your fingers towards each other and feel those energies. Again move your fingertips to and fro.

Exercise two

1. Ask a friend or your partner to participate. Standing with feet slightly apart, ask them to relax and breathe normally.

2. Stand in front of this person and hold the palms of your hands a body's width away from their head.

3. Slowly bring your palms in towards the head until you feel a change in the energy between your hands and their head.

4. Now slowly bring your palms down the body, continuing to trace the energy field around them.

5. Notice how far from the body it seems to project.

6. Be prepared for it to change.

7. Does it swell out or go in at some point? Does it feel cooler or warmer in places?

8. Repeat the process down the back and front.

9. How far above the top of the head does it extend?

10. Document your findings.

Exercise to Experience the Weight of the Aura

Select two people to stand on either side of you. They are going to try to pick you up by grasping your upper arm at the top and at the elbow. When they pick you up make sure that they do it in a way that lifts you straight up, rather than pushing you to one side.

First do it for practice to see how heavy you feel. Just stand normally thinking on nothing in particular. This is not about resisting. Sense how easy/difficult it is for them to pick you up. Now take some time to send your energy field upward. Focus on drawing your energy upwards, imagine being as light as a feather. When you have a good focus that you can sustain, ask them to try to pick you up.

Was it easier?

Now give yourself time to focus on increasing you connection with the ground. Grow roots from your fingertips and the bottom of your feet into the ground and deep into the earth. Concentrate on the strong and powerful energetic connection you have with the ground. When you have a very good focus, ask them to pick you up again.

Are you heavier and harder to pick up?

Balancing, Cleansing the Aura

Baths
One of the best ways of clearing your energy field if you have accumulated a lot of negative energy or have low energy due to an illness is to take bath in a combination of sea salt and baking soda. If you have trouble with low blood pressure, be

very careful as people have been known to faint in this bath. If you get dizzy, get out of the bath, and try it with cooler water. Soak for 20 minutes in the tub then lie in direct sunlight for 10-20 minutes to recharge your energy field. You will be surprised at how much cleaner you feel after this bath.

Aura Combing

Select a clean, clear quartz crystal and direct your intention into the crystal. This requires focus and clear thoughts. Start just above the head with faceted end towards the aura.

Make long sweeping movements towards the feet, always travelling a downwards direction. Hold the crystal well away from the energy field as you bring it up to commence the next sweep. Do at least ten long combing strokes.

This process can be beneficial before you go to sleep, during times of emotional stress, experiencing difficulties with another person or at the end of healing sessions.

Auric Brush

Another good way to groom your auric field is with the simple auric brush. It is like brushing your hair. One person stands with feet apart to shoulder width, arms at the sides, with eyes closed. The other begins at the front of the body. With fingers spread wide, reach up as far above the head of your partner as you can. Imagine that your fingers grow 6 inches longer than normal.

Begin now to use the elongated fingers of both hands as a brush. Make long and continuous sweeps from above the head down through the body, all the way to the ground. As you reach the ground, bell out the bottom of the field. Notice that your imaginary elongated fingers actually reach through the physical body. Make one long sweep down the body without stopping. Do not break the sweeping action. If you do, start over at the top of the head to prevent energy pile up.

Continue all round the body, covering the entire body till you reach the place where you started. Make sure you do not leave areas undone. This has a wonderful grounding effect.

The Aura Scan
Have your subject sit down comfortably on a chair. Begin to attune to your subject by placing your hands on their shoulders and breathe in a relaxed deep fashion. Stand to the side of your subject, far enough away so that you can extend your arms to sense their aura. Let your hands relax so that the fingers separate naturally. Start above the head and move slowly around and down to the feet.

Note any changes or discrepancies in the shape and feel of the aura. Be as open as you can to impressions you may pick up. Note where you feel the impressions to return to any part of the aura. Look for lumps, bumps, tears, holes, cold or hot spots and refer to the chart on this for healing techniques. Document your findings.

Use imagery if you prefer encompassing colors, shapes and sizes.

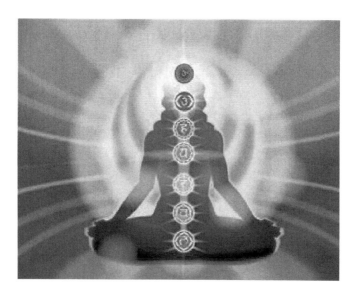

The Seven Sheaths

Ketheric Sheath

The Plane of Divinity

- ~ Position
- ~ Size, Structure and Color
- ~ Function/Purpose
- ~ Needs
- ~ Ketheric Sheath and the Endocrine System
- ~ Questions to Ask

PLANE	Spiritual
ASPECT	Higher concepts. Contains all the auric layers, past and present incarnation experiences.
ASSOCIATED WITH	Joy, power and universal love. Higher mind, knowing and integration of the spiritual and physical make-up.
SPIRITUAL AWARENESS	Service to humanity.
SOUL LEVEL	Divine Knowing. I know I am one with God. To be connected to and to understand the GREATER universal pattern.
CHAKRA	Crown — *Sahasrara*

INTERACTION WITH PHYSICAL BODY	Total integration of body, mind and spirit. Creates I am whole. My body is the temple of God.
BALANCED	Enlightenment, universal love and knowledge, perfection the end of the journey
IMBALANCED	Conditional, selfish, blocked from higher concepts

Position

This body extends 3 to 4 feet from the physical body depending on the person with the smaller tip between the feet and the larger end about 3 feet above the head. It can expand even more if the person is very energetic, particularly in service to humanity.

Size, Structure and Color

The outer edge appears much like an eggshell and appears to have a thickness of about a quarter to half an inch. Strong and resilient this sheath is resistant to penetration of other energies and protects the field just as an eggshell protects the chick. As the strongest of all the sheaths, it is highly structured and composed of tiny threads of gold-silver light which holds the whole form of the aura together. It contains the golden grid structure of the physical body and all the chakras. This sheath pulsates so fast that it almost shimmers and replicates a thousand golden threads.

Function/Purpose

This sheath regulates proper flow of energy out from the entire aura into the space beyond. It serves as a bridge between us and the cosmos and it holds within all the past life bands. The individual has little awareness of this level, as we live on the material plane, also it would be difficult for us to maintain this degree of consciousness. Nevertheless, it is sufficient for us to know that we are rooted into the universal life through this sheath, called the body of bliss.

Needs
The needs of this sheath are to experience serenity and to be connected to our divinity. This divinity brings a reason for being and the soul's purpose in this lifetime.

Ketheric Sheath and the Endocrine System
The Ketheric is associated with the pineal gland which acts as a link between this sheath and the physical body functions. It is the energy of faith. William James said, "Faith is the habitual center of human's personal energies."

Questions to Ask
What are the greater patterns threaded through my life?
What is the nature of the deeper hope that leads me?
Can I see how the pattern of my life has had a plan for my highest good?
What serene environment do I provide for myself?
How much time do I spend in serenity, being at one with God and the universe?
How much beauty and love do I see in everything?
How do I use faith in my life to generate my needs?

Celestial Sheath

The Plane of Intuition

> ~ Position
> ~ Size, Structure and Color
> ~ Function/Purpose
> ~ Needs
> ~ Celestial Sheath and the Endocrine System
> ~ Questions to Ask

PLANE	Spiritual
ASPECT	Higher mental aspects
ASSOCIATED WITH	Intuition, wisdom, devotion and spiritual mastery. Our own personal experience of spirituality and unconditional love.
SPIRITUAL AWARENESS	Spiritual nourishment to bring about spiritual experience.
SOUL LEVEL	To let go and let God. Divine love of self. Mastering lower thought processes.
CHAKRA	Brow *Ajna*
INTERACTION WITH PHYSICAL BODY	Balanced thought processes in alignment with Intuition. Creates materialization whole.
BALANCED	Spiritual intuition, wisdom, dignity, a sense of being connected to something higher.

IMBALANCED   Lack of self-worth, inability to envision or trust in the future, nightmares, irrational fear of the unknown.

Position
This body extends 2 and half to 3 and half feet from the physical body. It is the level through which we experience spiritual ecstasy.

Size, Structure and Color
The Celestial sheath appears as a shimmering light, composed mostly of pastel colors. This light has a gold-silver shine and opalescent quality, like mother of pearl sequins. Its form is less defined than the others and appears to be composed of light that radiates out from the body, like the glow around a candle. Sometimes this light is seen around the head and shoulders or emanating from the third eye area.

Function/Purpose
The primary function of this sheath is to receive higher inspirational thoughts and other mental phenomenon. In essence, this is about using our higher thought processes such as telepathy and intuition. Associated with the higher mind and the integration of our spiritual and physical make-up, we can reach this sheath through spiritual meditation and learning to use our spiritual eye (the third eye) rather than our physical eye.

Needs
The needs of this sheath are met by providing the spiritual environment in which to grow. This environment is one in which the intuitive mind can be developed. It also involves seeing with our non-physical eyes, non-judgmental attitudes and critical thoughts. When this is developed, dignity is of the

highest degree and people as a result feel dignified within your presence.

Celestial Sheath and the Endocrine System
This sheath is associated with the pituitary gland. The pituitary is the link between this sheath and the physical body functions. It is the energy of Imagination. Acting as the *third eye* of ancient mysticism, it is through this spiritual center that ultimate awakening comes and it is said one may enter the very presence of God through meditation and prayer.

Questions to Ask
What is the nature of my spiritual needs?
What is the nature of my spiritual feelings?
What environment do I provide for myself to nurture these spiritual needs?
Who are the people who assist in supporting my spiritual needs?
Are there some people I can let go of because they do not nurture my spiritual needs?
How much time do I allow myself each day to nurture my spiritual needs?
Do I trust my intuition and the guidance of my higher self?

Causal Sheath

The Plane of the Higher Self

~ Position
~ Size Structure and Color
~ Function/Purpose
~ Needs
~ Causal Sheath and the Endocrine System
~ Questions to Ask

PLANE	Spiritual
ASPECT	Higher emotional aspects
ASSOCIATED WITH	Truth and Inspiration. The power of the word in the creative process for Divine Will.
SPIRITUAL AWARENESS	'I will' according to the Higher Will. To speak and be in our truth.
SOUL LEVEL	Mastering the lower emotions. To align with the divine will within, to make the commitment to speak
CHAKRA	Throat *Vishuddha*
INTERACTION WITH PHYSICAL BODY	Balanced emotional states. Lower emotions transmuted into spiritual energy. Creates alignment.
BALANCED	Communication, families, truth, responsibility

IMBALANCED   Dishonesty, ignorance & isolation

Position
This sheath extends 2-3 feet from the body.

Size, Structure and Color
This sheath appears as clear or transparent lines on a cobalt blue background, much like an architect's blueprint. Each line represents the structure of the emotions.

Function/Purpose
This sheath is associated with higher will, the power of higher emotional thought, listening and taking responsibility for our actions. It holds the motivation or the plan for life that we would ideally love to live and is grounded in spiritual reality. The function and purpose of this sheath is to align the individual with Divine Will. On this level, the power of the word is very strong and carries with it a creative force. It means aligning oneself with the divine will within you and flowing with it.

Needs
The needs of the causal sheath is to speak ones truth and live by it. As this sheath deals with the higher emotions as opposed to the lower emotions it encompasses listening to the emotions via our spiritual higher selves which transmutes them. This raises our vibrations and creates a truth in alignment with the universal truths.

Causal Sheath and the Endocrine System
This sheath is associated with the thyroid and parathyroid glands and the link between this sheath and the physical body functions. It is the energy of power and is related to willpower. From the misuse of the power of words, may come

the condition known as hyper-thyroidism. When little effort is made to personal will, the opposite may occur, an imbalance known as hypo-thyroidism.

Questions to Ask

What is it that I need to say?

What is it I need to hear?

What is it that I need to say to close friends who may disagree with me?

What have I kept quiet about for many years?

Why haven't I expressed what I believe?

How do I use my expression?

Is it with loving words or with negative angry word?

How do I use the power of my will and words?

Astral Sheath

The Plane of Unified Love

~ Position
~ Size Structure and Color
~ Function/Purpose
~ Needs
~ Astral Sheath and the Endocrine System
~ Questions to Ask

PLANE	Astral
ASPECT	Bridge or doorway between planes
ASSOCIATED WITH	This layer connects us with higher dimensions acts as a doorway to the higher planes.
SPIRITUAL AWARENESS	How best to serve. Unconditional love, trans-personal love and harmony.
SOUL LEVEL	Interpersonal emotional life. Love, of humanity and compassion. To love and be loved by others in all forms.
CHAKRA	Heart *Anahata*
INTERACTION WITH PHYSICAL BODY	Yin/Yang balanced, spiritual metabolism of energies. I am loving. I am whole.
BALANCED	Renewal, harmony, balance, equality restoration, immunity, unconditional love

IMBALANCED   Isolation, stagnation, hardening, imbalance

Position
This body extends out about half to one foot from the physical body.

Size, Structure and Color
The astral body is formless and is composed of clouds of color infused with the rose light of love. When people fall in love, arcs of rose light can be seen between their hearts, and a beautiful rose color is added to the normal golden pulsations. Further to this, when people fall in love they grow cords out of the chakras that connect them to each other at various points on the body, for example the heart, mind or genital area. This is why broken relationships are just that, broken cords, and they carry with them a great deal of pain.

Function/Purpose
From this sheath, we interact with other people, animals, plants, inanimate objects, the earth, the sun, the stars and the universe as a whole. This is the center of love, and is the place of balancing the male/female energies. It holds the capacity to love and make connections between the physical individual and the subtle spiritual energies. When our heart center is open, the astral sheath acts like a bridge or doorway from the spiritual plane to the physical plane. If the doorway or bridge is not open, it prevents passage between our physical plane through to the spiritual plane and vice versa.

This sheath is where we master unconditional love. The heart area is the most abused and subject to closure than any other sheath. Relationships in particular, feeling pain, and the reluctance to feel pain and move through it places people in a position of fear and they can shut this area down. This produces bitterness, hurt and anger towards people.

Needs
The needs of the astral (heart) sheath are to give and receive love in all types of relationships. It needs loving interaction with your friends, family and associates as well as plants, animals and the universe. It needs unconditional love, forgiveness, and respect for all life and yourself along with non-judgmental criticisms to nurture yourself and humanity.

Astral Sheath and the Endocrine System
This sheath is associated with the thymus. The thymus is the link between this sheath and the physical body functions. The thymus gland is found behind the heart in the solar plexus area of the chest. Since the thymus gland is related to the heart, it is associated with love. Love opens all doors and at this center love is awakened, bringing with it consideration, unselfishness, sincerity and honesty.

Questions to Ask
Whom do I feel comfortable with and why?
Whom do I feel uncomfortable with and why?
Do I shut down when feeling hurt?
How can I remain open?
Do I feel resentment, bitterness or hurt over a past situation?
Am I open to the experience of love?
How do I demonstrate love, compassion forgiveness?

Mental Sheath

The Plane of Thought

~ Position
~ Size, Structure and Color
~ Function/Purpose
~ Needs
~ Mental Sheath and the Endocrine System
~ Questions to Ask

PLANE	Physical
ASPECT	Lower Mental aspect
ASSOCIATED WITH	Rational clarity that functions in harmony with our intuitive processes. Mental activity and sense of clarity.
SPIRITUAL AWARENESS	To understand the situation in a clear, linear, rational way utilizing all processes. Clear thinking used to implement love and will.
SOUL LEVEL	To express how we think about how we feel. How we manifest through our thoughts.
CHAKRA	Solar Plexus *Manipura*
INTERACTION WITH PHYSICAL BODY	Intellect, perception and cleansing and personal power. I am clear thinking. I am whole.

BALANCED   Intellect, security, optimistic, cleansing,
                        rational clear thoughts aligned with
                        intuitive processes.

IMBALANCED   Failing to learn from experiences, lack
                        of clarity, insecurity, negative thoughts,
                        toxicity.

Position

This body extends from 3-8 inches from the physical body. It
is composed of more finer substances than the emotional
body, all of which are associated with ideas and thoughts.

Size, Structure and Color

The mental layer is a structured body as it contains the structures of our ideas. It can be one of the hardest to see as human
beings are really just beginning to use their intellects in clear
ways. It usually appears as a bright yellow color, radiating
above the head and shoulders and extending around the
whole body. It expands and becomes brighter when the owner
is concentrating on mental processes. Thought forms shade
the color and can appear as blobs of varying brightness and
form. These are further superimposed with the person's
emotions. When this happens, it can create a double colored
effect of colors as the person's emotional level is connected to
the thought form. The clearer and well defined the thought,
the clearer and well defined the color. For example, a clear
thought form of love will show as clear green or pink where
as a confused or negative emotional thought form of love will
show as a muddy green or pink.

Function/Purpose

The mental sheath is a reflection of everyday thought patterns.
It reflects our mental nature, both negative and positive. The

primary function is much like a gathering device and helps us to develop the ability to use our mind in productive ways. It balances the lower sheaths by the power of our thoughts — positive thought. As energy follows thought, our development and evolution depends on how and where our thought is focused. With higher development, mental facilities bring new abilities, such as the ability to receive inspirational thoughts and intuitive ideas, telepathy and other mental phenomena.

Needs

The needs of the mental sheath relate to the mind and your need to understand and grow through situations in a clear, linear, rational way. The first step is to find and clear negative thoughts, beliefs, attitudes and judgments. They block the way to finding high solutions. Negative self-judgments are mental conclusions based on the negative way we feel about ourselves and these perpetuate negative feelings.

Mental Sheath and the Endocrine System

This sheath is associated with the spleen and pancreas and the link between this sheath and the physical body functions. It is the energy of judgment and joy. When we use our judgment incorrectly, we generate a flow of sorrow. This impedes our spiritual growth and ability to feel joy in our physical lives. Judgment and sorrow arise from mental processes and clog the energies of the spleen and pancreas interfering with the sweetness of life.

Questions to Ask

What are my negative ideas?

Where did I learn them from?

From whom?

Do I make more negative self-judgments about myself than others?

What are they?

Do I make them about others or other situations?

Can I identify negative processes, which interfere with a sweet flow in my life?

Emotional Sheath

The Plane of Emotion

~ **Position**
~ **Size Structure and Color**
~ **Function/Purpose**
~ **Needs**
~ **Emotional Sheath and the Endocrine System**
~ **Questions to Ask**

PLANE   Physical

ASPECT   Lower Emotional aspect

ASSOCIATED WITH   Energy and plenty — sexuality and creativity. All personal emotional relationships, emotional life and feelings. Expressing the full spectrum of our emotions.

SPIRITUAL
AWARENESS   Self acceptance and self love. This is where the inner child lives and loves.

SOUL LEVEL   To love and accept the self as we are. To reach our and embrace in whole feeling.

CHAKRA   Sacral *Svadhisthana*

INTERACTION WITH
PHYSICAL BODY   To relate to ourselves in a loving positive way honoring emotions in relation to physical health. I am real feeling. I am well.

BALANCED   Confidence, sociability, joy, plenty, creativity, partnership, inner child, able to complete emotional needs and master lower emotions.

IMBALANCED   Impoverished, not seeing to one's needs, lifeless, pessimistic, lonely, needy, unfeeling or unable to processes or master emotions.

Position

Like the etheric the emotional layer also surrounds and penetrates the physical body. Whilst the emotional sheath roughly follows the outline of the physical body it does not duplicate the physical body as does the etheric. Rather, it is more fluid and it moves in a continual fluid motion. It vibrates at a higher rate than both physical and etheric.

Size, Structure and Color

A healthy emotional sheath appears to be colored clouds of fine substance and extends 3-4 inches beyond the physical form. The color, shape and size vary according to the desires and emotions of the individual and whether these are felt negatively or positively. Clear and highly energized feelings such as joy, love and excitement show as bright and clear colors. Confused or angry feelings show as dark muddy colors. All colors can be found on this level and they flow along the structured lines of the etheric field. *Function/Purpose* This is the desire body, which experiences emotions — pleasure, pain, love and hate, and along with its appetites and moods, it shapes the physical. Every energy movement there correlates to a feeling you are having about yourself. Bright colors of cloud-like energy are associated with positive feelings. Darker, dirtier shades are associated with negative feelings. It is this energy, which attracts or repels other individuals. If we feel joyous, people are attracted to us; if we feel unworthy, others may ignore us.

Human emotions generate specific patterns of energy: hatred, lust, greed, desire, anger, love, devotion — each possess different vibrations. Its clarity and quality directly reflect the emotional responses. The emotional body reflects the interplay of emotions like a mirror. There is a constant play of energies as the emotional body mirrors all changes of mood and responds to the moods and vibrations of others. It mirrors without discrimination. Hence, this sheath can be dark, mirroring persistent ugly emotional states. The primary function therefore, is to express our feelings and love thereby transmuting these emotions to higher ones.

Needs

The needs of the emotional sheath is for self-acceptance and self-love. Issues on this level are self-esteem, worth or rejection. These are bad habits which need to be confronted directly. Most of us do not allow feelings about ourselves to flow. In particular, loving thoughts about ourselves are usually a low priority. We tend to criticize ourselves more readily than send ourselves love. The need of the emotional body is to allow emotions and feelings to flow whether they are good or bad. when we allow feelings about self to flow, whether they are negative or positive, the aura keeps itself balanced and the negative feelings and energies are released and transformed.

Emotional and the Endocrine System

This sheath is associated with the adrenals. The adrenals are the link between this sheath and the physical body functions. It is the energy of strength and zeal. The adrenal glands are the center of strength in times of stress, when it pours adrenaline into the bloodstream to aid us in fighting or fleeing. According to Edgar Cayce, the adrenals are also the storehouse of our emotional karma.

Questions to Ask
What are my needs with regard to accepting and loving self?
Which parts of my body do I dislike? Why?
How do I reject these parts?
Do I dislike myself when I do specific things?
What are these specific things?

Make a list of the ways that you reject yourself during any given day. Make a conscious effort to listen to yourself and replace any negative thoughts or words about yourself with positive ones.

Etheric Sheath

The Plane of the Physical

~ Position
~ Size, Structure and Color
~ Function/Purpose
~ Needs
~ Etheric Sheath and the Endocrine System
~ Questions to Ask

PLANE	Physical
ASPECT	Lower Physical aspect
ASSOCIATED WITH	The state between energy and matter. Reflecting the same structure as the physical body including all the anatomical parts and all the organs.
SPIRITUAL	Physical sensation; pleasure pain. Strength and vitality — personal survival.
SOUL LEVEL	I exist. Taking care of self. Physical/ personal survival. Simple physical comfort, pleasure and health. To have many wonderful physical sensations.
CHAKRA	Base *Muladhara*
INTERACTION WITH PHYSICAL BODY	Natural metabolism of energy which maintains the structure and function of the etheric body. I exist. I am whole. To enjoy a healthy body and all the physical sensations that go with it.

BALANCED   Energy, strength, vitality, and
                  grounding.

IMBALANCED   Lack of direction, no goals, no energy,
                  fear.

Position

Surrounding the physical body is the etheric body. It is a replica of the physical body and has the same structure, including all the anatomical parts and all the organs.

Size, Structure and Color

It is one of the first seen in aura practice and by far the brightest of a hazy-blue light. It extends 1 −2 inches beyond the physical form, however, it can extend up to 5 inches beyond the physical. If this is so, the intensity of light within it is far greater than normal.

The Etheric layer is very easy to feel and is referred to as the health aura or vital body, as patterns of disease appear first within the etheric form. It is made up of a kind of scaffolding of innumerable lines, employing various wavelengths and interactions with the cosmos. This scaffolding is composed of tiny energy lines. These tiny energy lines pulsate at about 15-20 cycles per minute. Where many lines cross a major chakra occurs, where only a few a minor. The etheric structure sets up the matrix for the cells to grow. This matrix is there before the cells grow.

Function/Purpose

The etheric forms part of the life support system and acts as a protective sheath for the physical form guarding it from all negative vibrations such as viruses and negative thoughts. The task of the etheric is to invigorate the physical one and pour into it transmuted energies from the earth and cosmos. It is an energy field, which interpenetrates, supports and conditions the physical body, nourishing the nervous system and the major organs, providing the energy needed for breathing, heartbeat and blood circulation. Within this level we feel all physical sensations, painful and pleasurable. There are direct correlations between the energy flow, field pulsation, and configuration in this level and the physical body. Wherever there is pain in your physical body, there is a direct correlation of dysfunction within the etheric sheath. The intensity of the pain reflects the intensity of dysfunction.

Needs
The etheric body has simple physical needs and requires energy boosts in order to maintain equilibrium, in particular where damage has occurred. This can be done through a combination of visualization, directed breathing and the laying on of hands. Energy can be sent directly to the etheric sheath or through the chakras. These two avenues direct colorful energy into the etheric body to strengthen it before directing energy onwards into the physical form. The etheric layer can be expanded and healed in this manner.

Etheric Sheath and the Endocrine System
This sheath is associated with the gonads. The gonads are the link between this sheath and the physical body functions. It is the energy of life and order. At the lowest level, if the gonads or sexual glands are used wholly on the sexual level and without control, they may create sexual perversions and unbridled sensuality. It is the place of cycles and those generated from spiritual order. As we strengthen the gonads we generate the energy of life and this strengthens our link to the etheric sheath.

Questions to Ask

What kind of environment do I need to best suit my physical needs?

Do I get enough sunlight and physical exercise?

Do I surround myself with reminders that will help all of my senses remember who I am?

Do I acknowledge my basic needs immediately?

What areas of my life do I not enjoy?

What senses are involved?

How do I strengthen and nurture my life cycles?

How does my physical life transmit order into my spiritual life?

The Nadis

["Nadis — three channels distributing pranic/chi energy to the chakras."]

- **Spiral Channels**
- **Pranayama**
- **Pranayama (Nostril Breathing) Technique**

Nadi is Sanskrit for *channel, stream or flow — energy in motion* and the nadis are the Sukshma channels through which prana (Sanskrit) or chi (Chinese) flow. There are said to be as many as 72,000 nadis. This prana or chi is considered a life force energy which flows to the chakras and then on to the physical body.

There is some debate between nadis and meridians, the system I discuss follows nadis and meridians as the same with the distinction that — three main nadis connect at the location of the major chakras and the 14 meridians which interconnect via the chakras and distribute prana or chi to the physical body.

Spiral Channels

["... a flowing river of life giving energy."]

The nadis consist of three spinal channels that weave around the chakra:

- **Shushumna** — Sanskrit for *channel, tube,* and originates at the base of the spine, (base chakra), and travels to the medulla oblongata at the base of the brain, (crown chakra). The chakras are strung along the inner column of Shushumna — a flowing river of life giving energy. It processes the inflow of energy from the etheric field of the aura. Shushumna has its main association with the governing meridian.

- **Ida** — Sanskrit for *comfort, introverted, moon,* and emerges up the left side of the base chakra. It represents the right hand side of the brain and represents female passive energy. This energy is distributed by the left nostril. Ida has its main association with the central meridian and processes the outflow of energy.

- **Pingala** — Sanskrit for *tawny, extroverted, sun,* and emerges up the right side of the base chakra and corresponds to the left hand side of the brain. This energy is distributed by the right nostril. Pingala has its main association with the central meridian and processes the outflow of energy.

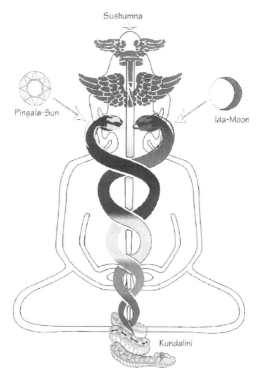

When we breathe in, we breathe through the Ida and Pingala. Where as the Ida and Pingala ascend and descend in a spiral fashion, the *Sushumna* moves up and down the spinal column. When our right and left breathes are equal in length and quality, via the Ida and Pingala breath, it becomes one balanced energy at the Sushumna Nadi in the center of the spine. The consequence of this is equilibrium and the state of homeostasis. This contributes to the maintenance of sustainable health as part of the holistic practice.

Pranayama

["... breathing is integral to the state of equilibrium or homeostasis."]

Pranayama, Sanskrit for *restraint of the prana or breath.* Composed of Prana — *life force or vital energy* and ayama — *to suspend or restrain.*

Many of us do not breathe in equal length or quality; most of us do not breathe via the nose. The simple act of breathing is integral to the state of equilibrium or homeostasis. A practice which assists the equal flow of breath is the practice of Pranayama.

The practice of Pranayama stimulates the Ida and Pingala Nadi and involves alternate breathing through left and right nostrils. This provides a flow of prana or life force energy to the Shushumna Nadi which then breathes energy into the chakras, meridians and the endocrine system and the vital organs of the human body.

The practice of Pranayama clears a foggy head, revitalises energy, calms the mind and nervous system, is useful in stressful situations, or if experiencing panic attacks and unifies the two hemispheres of the brain whilst providing life force energy into the chakras.

Yogic practices suggest, when the breath continues to flow in one nostril for more than two hours, as it does with most of us, it will have an adverse effect on our health. If the right nostril is involved, the result is mental and nervous disturbance. If the left nostril is involved, the result is chronic fatigue and reduced brain function.

Pranayama (Nostril Breathing) Technique

Using the Pranayama nostril breathing technique assists in balancing or harmonising the **endocrine system.** This process works directly with the hypothalamus and pineal. As energy is channelled through these centers it transmits through to the pituitary – thyroid – para-thyroids – thymus – adrenals – pancreas and gonads.

Pranayama nostril breathing assists in channelling clear energy into the aura which assists in balancing the subtle body in addition to providing clear energy through to the physical body.

1. Close the right nostril with your right thumb.

2. Take a slow, deep breath in through your left nostril, counting to eight. Slow down your in-breath so it takes eight seconds to fill your lungs.

3. Plug your left nostril (so both sides are now blocked) and hold your breath to a count of eight.

4. Now lift your thumb off your right nostril (keeping your left nostril plugged) and breathe out steadily, through your right nostril only, for a count of eight.

5. Do not pause at the end of the breath. Immediately start breathing in and breathe in through the right nostril to a count of eight.

6. Plug both sides and hold your breathe for a count of eight.

7. Now breathe out through your left nostril for a count of eight.

8. Start all over again, breathing in through your left nostril.

Breathe in and out as quietly as you can. This makes your breath slow and even.

Alternate nostril breathing should not be practiced if you have a cold or if your nasal passages are blocked in any way. Forced breathing through the nose may lead to complications. In Pranayama it is important to follow this rule: under no circumstances should anything be forced.

The Meridians

["Meridians — energy pathways distributing pranic/chi energy to the endocrine system and physical body."]

- **The 14 Meridian Channels**
- **Table of Meridian Characteristics**
- **The Meridians and the Five Elements**
- **Meridian Tapping Points**

Meridians or acupressure vessels are located throughout the body and constitute pathways which provide the flow of chi blood channels. As pathways of positive and negative energy they communicate to the body's systems and organs including the endocrine system.

Almost all points used in acupuncture and acupressure are situated along the 14 primary meridians. The meridians are classified yin or yang on the basis of the direction in which they flow. Yin energy is from the earth and flows upwards, from the feet to the torso and from the torso along the inside of the arms to the finger-tips. Yang energy is from the sun and runs downwards, from the fingers to the face or from the fact to the feet.

There is no actual beginning or end to this flow or movement; the meridians thus, represent a wheel. Moving around this wheel and following the meridian lines the flow follows this sequence on the body:

From torso to fingertip—fingertip to face—face to feet—feet to torso.

When this flow is unrestricted, the body has the opportunity to maintain homeostasis — generating a sustainable health. Any break in the flow is an indication that the chi flow is inadequate creating an imbalance and the body's vitality or energy diminishes. This can demonstrate as a malfunction in the body's organs or tissues and certainly a breakdown in homeostasis and equilibrium.

The 14 Meridian Channels

The 14 meridian channels carry energy into, through, and out of your body and correspond to specific human organs and to times of the day. Meridian flow is continuous and unbroken and moves in one definite direction from one meridian to the next in a well determined order providing a continuous flow of chi.

Traditional Chinese medicine shows us the principle of an internal set of instructions. Chi energy moves and circulates through out body in 24-hour cycles and are dictated by our organs. The chi spends two hours in each of the twelve organs.

Please note that just because the meridians are named according to the organs they pass through, it does not mean that they only correspond to these organs and their functions.

Table 2 Meridian Characteristics

Meridian	Physical Disturbances	Polarity
Stomach 7am – 9am	Stomach problems, abdominal pain, distension, edema, vomiting, sore throat, facial paralysis, upper gum toothache, nose bleeding, pain along the meridian	Yang↓ downward flow
Spleen 9am –11am	Problems of the spleen and pancreas, abdominal distension, jaundice, general weakness and sluggishness, tongue problems,	Yin ↑ upward flow

vomiting, pain and swellings along
the course of the meridian

Heart 11am – 1pm	Heart problems, dryness of the throat, jaundice, pain along the course of the meridian	Yin ↑ upward flow
Small Intestine 1pm – 3pm	Pain in the lower abdomen, sore throat, swelling or paralysis of face, deafness, pain along the meridian	Yang ↓ downward flow
Bladder 3pm – 5pm	Bladder problems, headache, eye diseases, neck and back problems, pain along the back of the leg	Yang ↓ downward flow
Kidney 5pm – 7pm	Kidney problems, lung problems, dry tongue, lumbago, edema, constipation, diarrhea, pain and weakness along the course of the meridian	Yin ↑ upward flow
Circulation Sex 7pm – 9pm	Poor circulation, angina, palpitation, diseases of the sexual glands and organs, irritability, pain along the course of the meridian	Yin ↑ upward flow
Triple Warmer 9pm – 11pm	Diseases of the thyroid and adrenal glands, ear problems, sore throat, abdominal distension, edema, swelling of cheek, pain along the meridian	Yang ↓ downward flow
Gall Bladder 11pm – 1am	Gall bladder problems, ear diseases migraine, hip problems, dizziness,	Yang ↓ downward

	pain along the meridian	flow
Liver 1am – 3am	Liver problems, lumbago, vomiting hernia, urination problems, pain pain in the lower abdomen and along the course of the meridian	Yin ↑ upward flow
Lung 3am – 5am	Respiratory diseases, sore throat, cough, common cold, pain in the shoulder and along the meridian	Yin ↑ upward flow
Large Intestine 5am – 7am	Abdominal pain, constipation, diarrhea, sore throat, toothache in the lower gum, nasal discharge and bleeding, pain along the course of the meridian	Yang ↓ downward flow
Central 7pm – 9pm	Diseases of the urogenital system, hernia, cough, breathing difficulties, breast problems	Yin ↑ upward flow
Governing 11am – 1pm	Spinal problems, mental disorders, fever, nose problems, headaches	Yin ↑ upward flow

As the body's energy bloodstream, the meridian system brings vitality and balance, removes blockages, adjusts metabolism, and even determines the speed and form of cellular change. Meridians affect every organ and every physiological system, including the endocrine, immune, reproductive, nervous, circulatory, respiratory, digestive, skeletal, and muscular.

The Meridians and the Five Elements

The five-element system is integral in traditional Chinese medicine and underscores the Chinese belief that human beings, both physically and mentally, are intertwined with nature. Each element governs a meridian and associated organ.

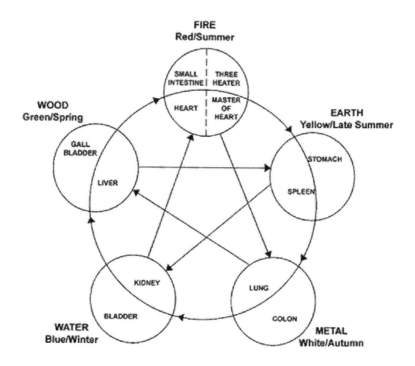

Fire Element

Yin Organ	Heart
Yang Organ	Small intestine
Odor	Scorched
Fortifies	Arteries
Taste	Bitter
Bodily Fluids	Sweat
Body	Pulse
Aperture	Tongue, Throat
Meridian	Small Intestine, Circulation Sex, Triple Warmer, Heart

Fire Meridians — *Chi* Channel

Hot, ascending, and light the fire element represents the heart (yin) and small intestine (yang) Meridians. The fire element also affects the complementary organ processes of the pericardium (yin) and the triple warmer, which is representative of the upper, lower, and middle parts of the body, as well as the circulation of fluids in these areas (yang).

Small Intestine (Si) — time of day 1– 3 pm
Muscles
~ Quadriceps
~ Abdominal Muscles

The Small Intestine Meridian starts from the tip of the little finger and crosses the palm and wrist. It runs upwards along the posterior side of the forearm until it reaches the back of shoulder to the bottom of the neck, then travels up the neck across the cheek then back to the ear.

Gland Meridian (Gd) — time of day 9– 11 pm (Triple Warmer)

Muscles

~ Teres Minor

~ Gastrocnemius

~ Satorius

~ Gracilis

~ Soleus

The Triple Warmer Meridian begins at the outer tip of the ring finger and goes along the back of the hand, wrist, forearm, and upper arm, until it reaches the shoulder region where it runs up the side of the neck, circles the ear and runs across the cheek to the outer end of the eyebrow.

Heart (H)— time of day 11 am – 1 pm

Muscles

~ Heart

~ Subscapularis

~ Subclavius

The Heart Meridian starts from the axilla (armpit) and runs along the inner side of the forearm, elbow and upper arm. It then crosses the inner side of the wrist and palm and ends at the inside tip of the little finger.

Circulation (C) — time of day 7– 9pm

Muscles

~ Gluteus Medius

~ Gluteus Maximus

~ Abductors Piriformis

Fire Addiction Tendencies:

Fire addictions tend to gravitate towards alcohol and psyche-delics and succumb to excesses of stimulation, flash, and color.

Common physical ailments are:

- Abdominal distension
- Angina, palpitations and hypertension
- Diseases of the sexual glands and organs
- Diseases of the thyroid and adrenal glands
- Ear problems
- Hyperglycemias
- Irritability
- Edema
- Poor circulation

Treatments to Bring About Balance:

- Balance Small Intestine — Heart — Circulation Sex and Triple Warmer Meridians

- Avoid concentrated or refined sugars, chocolate, purple fruits, cranberries, fats and fried foods

- Eat sources vitamin C, E, B and A — citrus fruits, green leafy vegetables, buckwheat, plenty of water, oily fish like salmon, salads with bitter leaves such as endive, radicchio and dandelion, dates and loganberry fruit, calcium, milk products, dolomite. Brewers yeast, legumes, nuts, eggs, yogurts, oysters, kelp

- Strengthen stomach muscles

- Avoid stimulant such as coffee and sugar and excessive spicy foods

Earth Element

Yin Organ	Spleen
Yang Organ	Stomach
Odor	Fragrant
Fortifies	Muscles
Taste	Sweet
Bodily Fluids	Saliva
Body	Muscle
Aperture	Lips, Mouth
Meridian	Stomach, Spleen

Meridians — Chi Channel

The Earth element relates to the stomach (yang) and the spleen (yin). The stomach begins the process of digestive breakdown, while the spleen transforms and transports the energy from food and drink throughout the body.

Stomach (S) — time of day 7– 9 am

Muscles

~ Levator Scpulae

~ Anterior Neck Flexors

~ Posterior Neck Extensors

~ Brachioradialis

~ Pectoralis Major Clavicular

The Stomach Meridian starts at the side of the nose, and passes through the inner corner of the eye to emerge from the lower part of the eye. Going downwards, it enters the upper gum and curves around the lips and lower jaw. It then turns upwards, passing in front of the ear, until it reaches the corner of the forehead where it crosses the neck, chest, abdomen and groin where it goes further downward along the front of the thigh and the lower leg, until it reaches the top of the foot. Finally, it terminates at the lateral side of the tip of second toe.

Spleen (Sp) — time of day 9– 11 am
Muscles
~ Latissmus Dorsi
~ Middle /Lower Trapezius
~ Opponens Pollicis Longus
~ Triceps

The Spleen Meridian begins at the big toe and runs along the inside of the foot crossing the inner ankle. It then travels along the inner side of the lower leg and thigh. It continues moving toward the chest and branches out to the axilla (armpit) and runs down the medial aspect of the torso parallel with the chest.

Earth Addiction Tendencies:
Earth addictions tend to gravitate towards foods, especially sweets. As a result, health problems tend towards digestive problems, spleen, and stomach organ system disorders.

Earth tends towards significant changes in their eating habits and they may fluctuate in weight, depending on their individual tendency to either halt or greatly increase their food intake.

Common physical ailments are:

- Abdominal pain
- Changing appetites
- Distension
- Indigestion
- Lethargy
- Muscle tenderness
- Nose bleeding
- Problems of the spleen and pancreas
- Stomach problems

- Upper gum toothache
- Water retention

Treatments to Bring About Balance:

- Balance stomach and spleen meridians

- Avoid sugars and sweets and emotional tension

- Eat sources of Vitamin B and A — wheat germ, whole grains, molasses, brewers yeast, yoghurt, kelp, green leafy vegetables, fish and hydrochloric acid

- Check for allergies and adrenals

- Avoid excess of tropical fruit such as bananas, pineapples and mangoes

- Avoid too many bakery items which puts too much strain on the digestion

- Avoid eating late or just before retiring for the night

Metal Element

Yin Organ	Lung
Yang Organ	Large intestine
Odor	Rotten
Fortifies	Skin & hair
Taste	Pungent
Bodily Fluids	Mucus
Body	Skin
Aperture	Nose
Meridian	Large Intestine, Lung

Meridians — Chi Channel

As a conductor the metal element includes the lungs (yin), which move vital energy throughout the body, and the large intestine (yang), which is responsible for receiving and discharging waste. Sadness, or grieving is the emotion which creates imbalance within this element.

Lung (L) — time of day 3– 5 am

Muscles

~ Serrartus (Anterior)

~ Anterior Serratus

~ Deltoids

~ Diaphragm

~ Coracobrachialis

The Lung Meridian branches out from the axilla (armpit) and runs down the medial aspect of the upper arm where it crosses the elbow crease. It continues until it passes above the major artery of the wrist, and emerges at the tip of the thumb.

Large Intestine (Li) — time of day 5– 7 am
Muscles
~ Quadrus lumborum
~ Hamstrings
~ Tensor Fascia Lata

The Large Intestine Meridian starts from the tip of the index finger and runs between the thumb and the index finger. It then proceeds along the lateral side of the forearm and the anterior side of the upper arm, until it reaches the highest point of the shoulder. From there, it travels externally upwards where it passes the neck and cheek, curves around the upper lip and crosses to the opposite side of the nose.

Metal Addiction Tendencies:
Metal addictions tend to gravitate towards tobacco and other smoking drugs.

Common physical ailments are:

- Abdominal pain
- Asthma
- Common cold
- Constipation and lower bowel disorders
- Cough
- Diarrhea
- Dry skin and hair
- Eczema and other skin disorders
- Nasal discharge and bleeding
- Pain in the shoulder
- Poor circulation
- Respiratory diseases
- Rhinitis
- Sensitive to climate

- Shallow breathing
- Sore throat
- Stiff joints and muscles
- Toothache in the lower gum

Treatments to Bring About Balance:

- Balance lung and large intestine meridians

- Avoid sugar and starchy foods

- Eat sources of Vitamin A, E and C — citrus fruits, honey, brewers yeast, yoghurt, green leafy vegetables, foods rich in metal i.e. foods like tofu, rice, raw onions, garlic, radish, turnip, kohlrabi, cinnamon, mint, rosemary, scallions, cloves, fennel, anise, dill, mustard greens, horseradish, mustard, basil, nutmeg are considered metal foods

- Drink plenty of water

- Avoid stuffy, polluted environments

Water Element

Yin Organ	Kidney
Yang Organ	Bladder
Odor	Putrid
Fortifies	Bones
Taste	Salty
Bodily Fluids	Urine
Body	Bones
Aperture	Ears
Meridian	Kidney, Bladder

Meridians — Chi Channel

Wet, descending, flowing, the water element represents the urinary bladder (yang), and the kidney (yin). The bladder receives, stores, and excretes urine. Water metabolism dissipates fluids throughout the body, moistening it, and then accumulating in the kidneys. The kidneys also store the essence, and serve as the root of yin and yang for the entire body. Fear and paranoia are the emotions, which create imbalance within this element.

Bladder (B) — time of day 3– 5 pm

Muscles

~ Peroneus Tertius

~ Sacrospinalis

~ Anterior/Posterior Tibial

The Bladder Meridian starts at the inner side of the eye and goes across the forehead to reach the top of the head then goes across the back of the head and divides into two branches. One branch crosses the center of the base of the neck and extends downwards parallel to the spine. Once in the lumbar region (bottom of the spine), it crosses the back of the shoulder and runs downward on the outside, which is adjacent and parallel to the inner branch. It continues down until it reaches the buttocks where two branches run across the back of thigh along different pathways that join at the back of the knee. The joint meridian then continues along the back of the lower leg, circles behind the outer ankle, runs along the outside of the foot and terminates on the lateral side of the tip of the small toe.

Kidney (K) — time of day 5– 7 pm

Muscles
~ Psoas
~ Iliacus
~ Upper Trapexius

The Kidney Meridian starts from the inferior side of the small toe. Crossing the middle of the sole and the arch of the foot, it circles behind the inner ankle and travels along the innermost side of the lower leg and thigh, across the pubic bone. It travels up over the abdomen upwards until it reaches the upper part of the chest (the inner side of clavicle).

Water Addiction Tendencies:

Water addictions tend to gravitate towards food related issues, but in this case with salty foods as well as sweets.

Common physical ailments are:

- Backache
- Chilliness
- Deteriorations of teeth and gum
- Dry tongue
- Eye diseases
- Hardening of the arteries
- Headache
- Kidney problems

- Loss of libido
- Lumbago
- Neck and back problems
- Edema, urinary and bladder
- Pain along the back of the leg

Treatments to Bring About Balance:

- Balance kidney and Bladder meridians

- Avoid coffee, purple fruits, cranberries, raw foods

- Eat sources of vitamin C, A, B and E — citrus, leafy green vegetables, wheat germ, Brewers yeast, legumes, nuts, eggs, papaya, yoghurts

- Drink plenty of water

- Consume calcium, milk products, dolomite

- To improve or alter an imbalance caused by a deficiency of water element I recommend naturally salty foods such as seaweed, miso soup and fish

- Find an exercise routine that will keep the knees and back strong

- Avoid raw/cold foods and icy fluids, which can have a sudden chilling effect

- Try to find the correct fluid intake, neither too much nor too little

Wood Element

Yin Organ	Liver
Yang Organ	Gall bladder
Odor	Rancid
Fortifies	Ligaments
Taste	Sour
Bodily Fluids	Tears
Body	Tendons
Aperture	Eyes
Meridian	Liver, Gall Bladder

Wood Meridians — Chi Channel

Strong, rooted — the wood element represents the liver (yin), and the gall bladder (yang).

The wood element allows for healthy balance in physical appearance and these are often well muscled individuals.

Liver Meridian — time of day 1– 3 am
Muscles
~ Pectoralis Major Sternal
~ Rhomboids

The Liver Meridian starts from the top of the big toe and goes across the top of the foot. After crossing the inner ankle, it continues to go upwards along the inner side of the lower leg and the thigh, until it reaches the pubic region. It goes up the abdomen and travels upwards over the liver area and up towards the chest finishing beneath the nipple area.

Gall Bladder Meridian — time of day 11 pm – 1 am.
Muscles
~ Anterior Deltoid
~ Popliteus/Shoulders

~ Sides of the body

The Gall Bladder Meridian starts from the outer corner of the eye and weaves back and forth at the lateral side of the head. After curving behind the ear, it reaches the top of the shoulder and crosses the lateral side of rib cage and abdomen, until it ends up at the side of the hip. It then runs toward the lateral side of the thigh and lower leg. After crossing the ankle, it goes over the foot to reach to the tip of the fourth toe.

Wood Addiction Tendencies:
Wood element addictions tend to gravitate towards stimulants, sedatives, alcohol, opiates, and amphetamines.

Common physical ailments are:

- Balance, coordination symptoms
- Dizziness
- Ear diseases
- Fatigue: worse early morning
- Gall bladder problems
- Gallstones
- Headaches or migraine
- Heavy menses, dysmenorrheal
- Hepatitis and other liver organ system disorders
- Hernia
- High blood pressure
- Hormonal imbalance
- Insomnia - end of night
- Lumbago - low lumbar, radiate to hips, sacroiliac
- Muscular problems: cramps, tendonitis, muscle spasms
- Nerve inflammations
- One sided symptoms
- Physical problems with eyes

- Urination problems
- Weak nails

Treatments to Bring About Balance:

- Balance gallbladder and liver meridians

- Avoid fats and fried foods, sweets, alcohol, caffeine, carbonated drinks

- Eat sources of Vitamin A — carrots and green leafy vegetables

- Drink plenty of water to flush out toxins from the organs

- Relaxation techniques

Endocrine Meridian

The Endocrine Meridian begins at the outer tip of the ring finger and goes along the back of the hand, wrist, forearm, and upper arm, until it reaches the shoulder region where it runs up the side of the neck, circles the ear and runs across the cheek to the outer end of the eyebrow.

To stimulate, run your hand from the ring finger, as if to trace along an imaginary dotted line along the back of the arm up over the shoulder, up the side of the neck, past the cheek side of the ear and across the cheek to the outer edge of the eye. Do this three times.

Many complementary therapists provide professional assistance for the meridians. For example: Kinesiologists, Chinese Medicine, Reflexologists, Naturopaths, Acupuncturists.

Meridian Tapping Points

Understanding the meridian system is not difficult and we can assist the flow of energy throughout our bodies with these understanding and gentle tapping techniques.

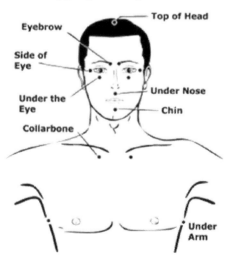

As a daily practice, tap these points to stimulate the meridians towards balancing the endocrine system and gaining a kick-start to the day.

Balancing Yin and Yang Meridian Flow

1. Crown of Head — Tap gently with the flat of your hand on the mid-line at the top of your head, about 3 centimeters forward from the actual crown. Tapping this point stimulates all yang meridians, distributing energy downward to lower parts of your body.

2. Inner Wrist — Slap sharply 3 fingers above your inner wrist crease on each forearm to stimulate all upper yin channels. The polarity of yin energy is opposite to yang. Yin meridians tend to distribute energy upwards. The inner wrist points send yin energy to the upper part of your body.

3. Inner Ankle — Slap sharply 4 fingers above the point of your ankle on the inside of each leg. From this point, you stimulate all Lower Yin meridians. Your inner ankle points send yin energy upward, thus serving all lower areas of your body. This finishes balancing yang and yin polarities.

The Chakras

["Chakras — energetic vortices located along the major meridians."]

- **Chakra Theories**
- **Power to Heal**
- **Chakras in Relation to Other Systems**
- **Table 2 Chakras, Associated Glands, Meridian**
- **Individual Chakras**
- **Table 3 Chakra and Meridian Correlations**

Chakra is a Sanskrit for *wheel* which is symbolic of life and cyclical patterns and the principles of nature. They play an important role in the human body as they are responsible for processing the energies within the body. Essentially they can be viewed as transmission stations and a connection between the physical and subtle world of energies. Chakras are also believed to be spiritual blueprints and carry information regarding one's entire cycle.

Chakra Theories

["… by harnessing the power therein one can advance healing.']

History is dotted with discussions re these ancient symbols — Pilo (Jewish Philosopher) along with Aristotle, Paracelsus revered them as major energy cores with the ability to assist healing. In much the same way, eastern philosophy embraces the Chakras as a way of healing, and by harnessing the power therein one can advance healing. The notion of the Chakras is not exclusive to ancient seers or eastern philosophies. The system of power vortices or energy cores is evident through the calculations and measurements found in great landmarks such as the

Pyramids, Stonehenge, Gothic cathedrals, Egyptian temples, Buckingham Palace, the Vatican, Taj Mahal, Kremlin, Washing DC, Cologne Cathedral, and The Pantheon.

David Tansley has this to say about chakras in his book *Radionics and the Subtle Anatomy of Man:*

"A chakra may be defined as a focal point for the reception and transmission of energies. These energies can originate from a variety of sources, some cosmic, others from the collective unconscious of a nation or humanity..."

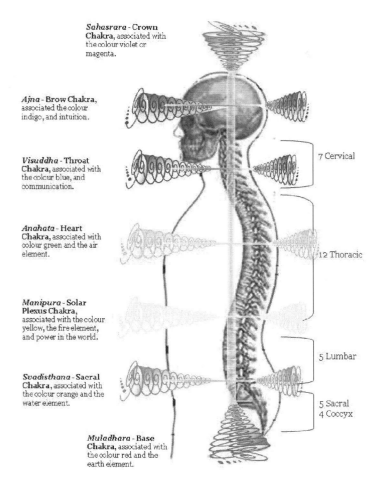

Sahasrara - **Crown Chakra,** associated with the colour violet or magenta.

Ajna - **Brow Chakra,** associated the colour indigo, and intuition.

Visuddha - **Throat Chakra,** associated with the colour blue, and communication.

Anahata - **Heart Chakra,** associated with colour green and the air element.

Manipura - **Solar Plexus Chakra,** associated with the colour yellow, the fire element, and power in the world.

Svadisthana - **Sacral Chakra,** associated with the colour orange and the water element.

Muladhara - **Base Chakra,** associated with the colour red and the earth element.

7 Cervical

12 Thoracic

5 Lumbar

5 Sacral
4 Coccyx

The chakras have three main functions:

1. To vitalize the physical body
2. To bring about the development of self-consciousness
3. To transmit spiritual energy in order to bring the individual into a state of spiritual being

Power to Heal

Each major chakra in the human body is a center of swirling energy positioned at one of seven points, from the base of the spine to the top of the head. Where the meridians deliver their energy to the organs, the chakras bathe the organs in their energies. At the center of each chakra, in its deepest point, there is a stem-like channel that extends to the spine and merges with it. The chakras are connected to the Sushumna Nadi via these stems, which provides each chakra with living and vital energy.

On a subtle body level, chakras filter energy from the environment via the aura into the meridians into the physical body level and onto the systems of the body and the major organs. Each chakra supplies energy to specific organs. A sensitive practitioner's hand held over a chakra may resonate with pain in a related organ, congestion in a lymph node, subtle abnormalities in heat or pulsing, areas of emotional turmoil, or even tune into a stored memory that might be addressed as part of the healing process.

The state of each chakra reflects the health of a particular area of your body. It also reflects your psychological, emotional and spiritual wellbeing. Every thought and experience you've ever had in your life is filtered through the chakra databases. Each event is recorded into your cells. In other words, your esoteric biography becomes your biology. When chakra energy is blocked or misdirected, emotional and physical illness can arise.

Chakras in Relation to Other Systems

Where the endocrine system is the physical body's Personal Tuning Fork the chakras can be considered the subtle body's Personal Tuning Fork.

Chi from the meridians flows into the chakras and this energy spirals up and into the auric field. Each chakra correlates with an endocrine gland, auric layer and a meridian channel. Just as earth power spots fall upon ley lines so too the chakras fall upon meridian channels, each meridian will have a primary chakra correlation and a secondary correlation.

Table 2 Chakras, Associated Glands, Meridian

Sahasrara — Crown Chakra

Endocrine Association	Associated with the Hypothalamus and Pineal Gland
Meridian Association	Governing, Triple Warmer Meridians
Auric Layer	Ketheric

Ajna — Third Eye Chakra

Endocrine Association	Associated with the Pituitary Gland
Meridian Association	Governing Meridian
Auric Layer	Celestial

Vishuddha — Throat Chakra

Endocrine Association	Associated with the Thyroid and Para-thyroids Glands

Meridian Association	Central Meridian
Auric Layer	Causal

Anahata — Heart/Emotions Chakra

Endocrine Association	Associated with the Thymus Gland
Meridian Association	Lung, Heart Meridians
Auric Layer	Astral

Manipura — Solar Plexus Chakra

Endocrine Association	Associated with the Pancreas and Adrenal Glands
Meridian Association	Large Intestine, Small Intestine, Circulation Sex, Meridians
Auric Layer	Mental

Svadhisthana — Sacral Chakra

Endocrine Association	Associated with the Spleen and the Adrenals
Meridian Association	Stomach, Gall Bladder, Liver Meridians.
Auric Layer	Emotional

Muladhara — Base Chakra

Endocrine Association	Associated with the Gonads and Adrenal Medulla
Meridian Association	Kidney, Circulation Sex and Bladder Meridians

Auric Layer   Etheric

Individual Chakras

Sahasrara

- ~ Spiritual Message
- ~ Life Issues
- ~ Sahasrara and the Glands
- ~ Sahasrara, the Aura, and the Soul
- ~ An Out of Balance Sahasrara

Sahasrara, pronounced: *Suh-us-ra-ar*, is Sanskrit for *Thousand Spoked Wheel*, and is the highest yogic center.

Generically it is known as the crown chakra and is symbolised by a lotus with a thousand petals and is associated with the color violet or magenta. Its spiritual function is spiritual wisdom and faith.

Located in the brain, it is the chakra of consciousness, enlightenment, dynamic thought, truth and oneness. The crown chakra finds outward expression through the right eye, and the upper brain.

Spiritual Message

Knowing through the higher mind, an encompassed love for all mankind as an integrated whole.

Life Issues

The life issues associated with this chakra involve the ability to trust life, values, ethics, courage, humanitarianism, selflessness, ability to see the larger pattern, faith, inspiration, spirituality and devotion.

Sahasrara's sacred truth is to live in the present moment and achieve a personal relationship with the Divine. All physical, psychological and emotional illusions or fears need to be removed from your life. Let go of the past, do not anticipate the future and live in the presence of the Divine.

Sahasrara and the Glands

Sahasrara (Crown) is connected to the pineal gland and also connects to the central nervous system via the hypothalamus. The thalamus bears a key role in the physical basis of consciousness. The pineal gland produces melatonin and this hormone affects the other glands in the endocrine system and mirrors the crown chakra's relationship with the other chakras. It also produces trace amounts of the psychedelic chemical dimethyltryptamine. Philosophers and spiritual adepts have shrouded the pineal in mystery and speculation for centuries. Ancient Greek physician Galen, (Claudius Galenus of Pergamum (131-201 AD), said the pineal was a regulator of thought and that the soul was anchored there.

The Chinese liken the Pineal to the tiger force, which marries with the pituitary dragon force. The pineal releases a spiritual essence representing the spiritual will to be a soul.

Sahasrara, the Aura, and the Soul

Sahasrara correlates with the ketheric body of the aura. The ketheric body controls and influences the area of consciousness known as the spiritual realm. Within this body exists our spiritual life as an evolutionary imprint or reflection from the soul and reveals both the spiritual quality of the individual and the state of consciousness. The size, variation in color, speed, rhythm as well as development of the interconnections with other centers, all indicate the quality and character of the whole personality and the strength of its connection with innermost self.

This is the center in which we normally exit during sleep. The size of its core, as well as the other characteristics indicates the individual's ability to expand in consciousness. In other words, this chakra reveals the stage of conscious evolution in the individual. When the crown and brow centers are open and active, clairvoyance is possible along with the ability to meditate.

An Out of Balance Sahasrara

Possible physical areas affected by an out of balance chakra:
Exhaustion, energetic disorders, epilepsy, pineal gland, right eye, muscular system, skeletal system and skin.

Possible spiritual/emotional areas affected by an out of balance chakra:
The crown chakra is about wisdom and being one with the world and its function is *unity of consciousness*. When this chakra is open and balanced, it generates unprejudiced and a developed awareness of the world and self.

If it is under-active, one will be unaware of spirituality and thinking process will be rigid or 'black and white'. This can generate feelings of separation from the universe, lack of bliss, an inability to see larger picture, spiritual depression, and inability to surrender to flow of life.

When over-active, it can generate feelings of disconnection from earth and reality and extreme sensitivities to light, sound and other environmental factors. One will tend towards over intellectualizing rather than connecting to heart centers for wisdom. There is also the tendency towards being addicted to spirituality thus ignoring the bodily needs.

Ajna

~ Spiritual Message
~ Life Issues
~ Ajna and the Glands
~ Ajna, the Aura, and the Soul
~ An Out of Balance Ajna

Ajna, pronounced: *arj-na,* and is Sanskrit for command center, direction and injunction.

Generically it is known as the third eye chakra, is symbolized by a lotus with two petals, and is associated with the color indigo. Its spiritual function is connection with higher self and clairvoyance.

Located at the base of the brain it is the chakra of time and awareness and of light and is linked to the pituitary gland which releases hormones influencing body chemistry.

Spiritual Message

Intuitional thinking and conceptual ideas through the ability to visualize and seek higher answers.

Life Issues

The life issues associated with this chakra involve self-evaluation, truth, intellectual abilities, feelings of inadequacy, openness to the ideas of others, ability to learn from experience, emotional intelligence.

Ajna's sacred truth is to seek only the truth and continually search for the difference between truth and illusion, the two forces present themselves with every moment. The essence is, to trust what you cannot see more than what you can see.

Ajna and the Glands

There has been much discussion and research regarding the

third-eye and associated glands. Earlier civilizations considered the third-eye to be an organ. Ancient doctrines talk of beasts with three eyes. Helena Blavatsky's *The Secret Doctrine* talks of *"four-armed male-females* (hermaphrodites) *human creatures with one head, yet three eyes. The third eye was at the back of the head ..."*

Vera Stanley Alder in *The Fifth Dimensions* discussed similar concepts: *"the Pineal and the Pituitary is male and female aspects of the androgynous brain ..."* talked of the harmonious blend of the two glands using the term, to marry, and in this state an individual achieves a direct link to the Christ Consciousness, gaining perception and wisdom beyond the five senses.

In Traditional Chinese Medicine, similar theories espouse the third-eye along with its gland the pituitary representing the dragon feminine, a creative force inspired by higher consciousness and imagination. The energy gathers momentum and spirals forward into a union with the spirit in the pineal. This union or marriage is the power-source and controller of the endocrine orchestra. In a balanced state, the two in harmony, the individual is successful and in inspirationally enthusiastic.

Ajna, the Aura, and the Soul

Ajna correlates with the celestial body of the aura and is of the spiritual realm. It is the body which holds our individualistic future and is also our access to the future. This is where we actively focus our mental and intuitive energy.

This chakra is concerned with the integration of new ideas and experience with the capacity of organisation. It is the seat of the mind and the point through which the higher self begins to command the lower will once a certain stage of development is attained. Prior to this, where the individual exerts little or no control over communications from non-physical beings, they are merely psychic, unable as yet to communicate with the higher planes of consciousness.

If the etheric brow is well developed and its interconnections with its astral counterpart are open and active, then clairvoyance or a higher order is possible. When it is interconnected, primarily with the throat center, this indicates an active use of the creative imagination.

An Out of Balance Ajna

Possible physical areas affected by an out of balance chakra:
Glaucoma, headaches, neurological problems, cerebellum, nose, pituitary, central nervous system, left eye, brain, nervous system, eyes, ears, nose, pineal gland, hemorrhage, stroke, neurological disturbances, blindness, deafness, full spinal difficulties, learning disabilities, seizures.

Possible spiritual/emotional areas affected by an out of balance chakra:
The Third Eye chakra is about insight and visualization. Its function is connection with higher self and when open you will experience intuition, and be in touch with dreams.

When under-active there is a tendency towards inability to think for self or trust in ones ability to be clear about what is best. There can be rigidness in thinking, relying on beliefs too much and becoming confused easily. This can generate feelings of: disconnection from soul, inability to focus and stay centerd, lack of intuition, rigid beliefs, overanalyzing. In excessive cases hallucinations are possible. When over-active there is a tendency towards living in a world of fantasy and this can generate feelings of oversensitivity, and feeling spaced out.

Vishuddha

~ Spiritual Message
~ Life Issues
~ Vishuddha and the Glands
~ Vishuddha, the Aura, and the Soul
~ An Out of Balance Vishuddha

Vishuddha, pronounced: vish-ud-dha, and is Sanskrit for pure and cleansing.

Generically known as the throat chakra and is symbolized by a lotus with sixteen petals and associated with the color blue. Its spiritual function is creativity and communication. It is the center for sound, communication, speech, writing and thought expression and growth being a form of expression.

Spiritual Message

Using the power of the word by speaking truth. Affirming things into manifestation, listening and taking responsibility for actions.

Life Issues

The life issues associated with this chakra involve choice and strength of will, personal expression, following your dream, using personal power to create, addiction, judgment, criticism, faith, knowledge, capacity to make decisions.

Vishudda's sacred truth is to surrender personal will to divine will. Our every choice, thought and feeling has biological, environmental, social, personal and global consequence. Actions motivated by personal will that trusts divine authority, give you the richest power.

Vishuddha and the Glands

Located in the throat it is linked to the thyroid and parathyroid glands. The throat chakra divides into male and female, dual energies of thyroids and parathyroids representing active intelligence and expression. Here, duality appears and the separation of male and female into right and left sides continues down the body, beginning in the right eye — male pineal and left eye female pituitary forces. The thyroid is the focal point for higher creative energies and is the polar opposite of the gonads, the sexual reproductive glands.

Vishuddha, the Aura, and the Soul

Vishudda correlates with the etheric body of the aura and it is the first in the spiritual realm, as the template for the physical body, the spiritual matrix for our physical being. Those who use their voice a great deal, singing, public speaking, musicians and composers have a brighter faster moving chakra. It is the creative aspect of the self and is transmitted through the brow chakra.

The throat center has links with the crown and brow chakras in certain states of expanded consciousness, and is especially important with respect to the interconnections between the mental and the etheric fields.

An Out of Balance Vishuddha

Possible physical areas affected by an out of balance chakra:
Asthma, neck problems, lungs, hypoactive thyroid, alimentary canal, vocal cords, trachea, neck vertebrae, mouth, teeth, gums, jaw, esophagus, parathyroid, throat problems, mouth ulcers, gum difficulties, TMJ, scoliosis, laryngitis, swollen glands.

Possible spiritual/emotional areas affected by an out of balance chakra:
The throat chakra is about self-expression and talking. Its function is creativity and communication and when it is open, we will be able to express ourself, and that includes ideas, thoughts, feelings, creativeness or artistic abilities and higher wisdom.

When this chakra is under-active there is a tendency towards inability to express through speaking, holding on and back, introversion and shyness. This can generate feelings of excessive rationality, lack of creativity, inability to find a life vision, lack of communication, unvoiced feelings. Not speaking the truth may block this chakra.

If this chakra is over-active, there is a tendency towards talking too much, which can distance others or generate feelings of criticism from others.

Anahata

~ Spiritual Message
~ Life Issues
~ Anahata and the Glands
~ Anahata, the Aura, and the Soul
~ An Out of Balance Anahata

Anahata, pronounced: *arn-a-hud-a*, and is Sanskrit for unstruck sound, because the unstruck sound is the sound of silence, and Anahata is where the silence of your divine consciousness resides.

Generically it is known as the heart/emotions chakra, and is symbolized by a lotus with twelve petals and is associated with the color green. Its spiritual function is — love, equilibrium, and wellbeing.

Spiritual Message

Compassionate love, being able to give and receive forgiveness and God's love.

Life Issues

The life issues associated with this chakra involve love, hatred, bitterness, grief, anger, jealousy, inability to forgive, self-centeredness, fears of loneliness, commitment and betrayal, compassion, hope trust, ability to heal yourself and others.

Anahata's sacred truth is love and divine power. Emotional energy — love — is the central power point and true motivator of your body, mind and spirit.

Anahata and the Glands

The thymus is located above the heart and produces lympho-cytes, which form a vital part of the body's immune response. This quality relates the thymus to the healing properties of the

176

heart chakra.

David Tansley say about chakras in his book *Radionics and the Subtle Anatomy of Man*, says the thymus is *"related to the life thread anchored in the heart, in this chakra of LOVE in the heart center. Here the higher the consciousness and the more illuminated one's love consciousness the more effective is the protective immune center. When children are loving and open, this center functions well, and when we close down in adult life, the gland atrophies and loses it ability to protect."*

Anahata, the Aura, and the Soul

Anahata correlates with the astral body of the aura and is the first level beyond three-dimensional reality, that experiential level just above the physical, emotional and intellectual planes. The astral is the level of consciousness that bridges the dimensions of matter and spirit. It is the plane to which we travel when we sleep.

This chakra is linked to the higher dimensions of consciousness and with ones sense of being and has a close relationship with the crown chakra. The heart center registers the quality and power of love in the individual's life. When a person has transformed personal desires and passions into a wider and universal compassion and love of his fellows, the heart becomes the focus of energies, which were formerly concentrated in the solar plexus.

In meditation, it is encouraged to focus on the heart center, in order to strengthen its connection with the core of the crown chakra. This brings about a state of true balance in the body, for the heart center is really the point of integration in the whole chakra system. The heart center acts as a primary factor in spiritual transformation.

An Out of Balance Anahata

Possible physical areas affected by an out of balance chakra:
Cancer, high blood pressure, heart problems, thymus, blood, involuntary muscles, center of the chest, heart and circulatory system, lungs, arms and hands, ribs/breasts, diaphragm, thymus gland, asthma/allergy, bronchial pneumonia, upper back, shoulder pain, breast cancer.

Possible spiritual/emotional areas affected by an out of balance chakra:
The heart chakra is about love, kindness and affection. Its function is love, equilibrium, and emotional wellbeing and when it is open, you will be compassionate, empathetic and friendly. An open heart chakra means we will be able to remain open when hurt or angry. Bringing with it the ability to find it easier to work at harmonious relationships.

When under-active there is a tendency towards being cold and distant. The heart will be closed particularly when hurt or angry. This can generate feelings of resentment, anger, depression, lonliness and suppressed feelings.

When over-active there is a tendency towards suffocating people with your love and love from neediness and selfish motives. This can generate feelings of service to others at expense of self, martyr syndrome.

Manipura

~ Spiritual Message
~ Life Issues
~ Manipura and the Glands
~ Manipura, the Aura, and the Soul
~ An Out of Balance Manipura

Manipura, pronounced: *mani-poor-a*, and is Sanskrit for city of jewels, because it has so many conduits of pranic energy intersecting there, and because it is the place where the fires of digestion burn.

Generically it is known as the solar plexus chakra, and is symbolised by a lotus with ten petals and is associated with the color yellow. Its spiritual function is social survival, self-esteem, power and control. Manipura is located above the navel and linked to the pancreas, the outer adrenal glands, and the adrenal cortex.

Spiritual Message
Personal power and how to take care of self on an emotional and mental level.

Life Issues
The life issues associated with this chakra involve trust, fear, intimidation, self-esteem, self-confidence, self-respect, ambition, courage, ability to handle crisis, care of yourself and others, sensitivity to criticism, personal honor, fear of rejection and looking foolish, physical appearance anxieties, strength of character.

Manipura's sacred truth is to honor oneself. Be mature and honorable in the relationship you have with yourself and accept responsibility for the person you have become.

Manipura and the Glands

The pancreas rests in the dark cauldron of the solar plexus center. It is centered where the diaphragm valve releases or holds a vault of emotions. When this valve opens it allows natural expression and cleansing of suppressed energies. This is a vital process towards holistic health as the act of suppression not only pollutes the physical and spiritual systems it drains vital energies.

It is here, through the naval along with the pancreas that the positive fiery functions provide the earthly foundation for the mental and spiritual life.

Manipura, the Aura, and the Soul

This chakra is the seat of the lower will or ego and is the point of focus for all desires of the lower self. It fluctuates in rhythm, hyperactivity and disturbances in the color patterns of this center indicates a person who over-identifies with his emotions and cannot easily control his feelings.

This chakra is most important in respect to the connection with the emotional field, since it is at this point that the astral energy enters the etheric fields. Consequently, it is the center through which the vast majority of individuals express themselves. It is also closely linked to the heart and the throat chakras.

In the life of an ordinary person, the solar plexus is probably the most important and active of all the chakras since it is very much involved with the emotional life. This is the center most used by trance-mediums and is involved in many less developed types of clairvoyance.

An Out of Balance Manipura

Possible physical areas affected by an out of balance chakra:
Diabetes, digestive illness, hypoglycemia, ulcers, abdomen, stomach, upper intestines, liver, gallbladder, kidney, spleen, middle spine behind the solar plexus, arthritis, gastric or

duodenal ulcers, colon/intestinal problems, pancreatitis, diabetes, chronic or acute indigestion, anorexia, bulimia, liver dysfunction, hepatitis, adrenal dysfunction.

Possible spiritual/emotional areas affected by an out of balance chakra: The solar plexus chakra is about assertion. Its function is social survival, self-esteem, power and control. When it is open, we feel in self-control empowered and confident with high self esteem. When under-active there is a tendency towards passiveness, indecisive and not getting what we want. This can generate feelings of low self-esteem; a need to live up to others' expectations.

When over-active there is a tendency towards domineering behavior and this can generate feelings of over inflated ego, overly competitive, stored rage.

Svadhisthana

~ Spiritual Message
~ Life Issues
~ Svadhisthana and the Glands
~ Svadhisthana, the Aura, and the Soul
~ An Out of Balance Svadhisthana

Svadhisthana, pronounced: *Swar-dish-tarn-ya*, and is Sanskrit for ones self, ones own seat or abode.

Generically it is known as the sacral chakra, and is symbolized by a lotus with six petals and is associated with the color orange. Its spiritual function is genetic survival, relationships, emotional self, physical and material desires. The potential for life in the ovaries is mirrored in the drives of the sacral chakra. Located between the navel and pubic bone it is linked to the gonads — testicles or the ovaries — which produce the various sex hormones involved in the reproductive cycle, and can cause dramatic mood swings. The energies of the ovaries link with the sacral chakra.

Spiritual Message
The emotional aspects, sensuality and the home of the inner child.

Life Issues
The life issues associated with this chakra involve fear of loss of control, or being controlled, through events such as addiction, rape, betrayal, impotence, financial loss, or abandonment along with the ability to take risks, personal identity, blame, guilt, money, sex, power, control, creativity, ethics, honor in relation-ships, decision-making, power to rebel.

Svadhisthana's sacred truth is to honor one and other. Every relationship we develop, from casual to intimate, helps us to become more conscious. No union is without spiritual value.

Svadhisthana and the Glands

The gonads manifest the active counterpart of pineal or pituitary, whether the person becomes dominant male of female, the concerns itself with sexual reproduction and of the species preservation. If energies are concentrated underlying lust, loss of mental and spiritual consciousness results and the person is burdened in the physical life, to the detriment of developing the higher centers. This energy is also related to the will to create on the physical plane closely linked to thyroid control.

Svadhisthana, the Aura, and the Soul

Svadhisthana correlates with the emotional body of the aura and all emotions are processed here and are under the dominion of this second center.

When balanced it brings a sense of self-confidence and creativity and the imagination is used constructively and sexual energy brings a sense of completeness. In a woman this chakra includes the womb and can be seen emanating from the physical form.

An Out of Balance Svadhisthana

Possible physical areas affected by an out of balance chakra:
Bladder problems, frigidity, gall and kidney stones, reproductive organs, vaginal cancer, prostate cancer, pelvic disease, lower abdomen to navel, large intestine, lower vertebrae, appendix, bladder, arthritis, chronic lower back or hip pain, sciatica, urinary problems, fibroids, menopause severity.

Possible spiritual/emotional areas affected by an out of balance chakra:
The sacral chakra is about feeling and sexuality and when open generates intimacy and well balanced sexuality. Its function is

related to genetic survival, relationships, emotional self, physical and material desires. When it is open, feelings flow freely, and will be expressed without excessive emotions or over-emotional outbursts.

When under-active there is a tendency towards being unemotional and being closed to people emotionally. This can generate fear of intimacy, fear of abandonment, disassociated from sexuality, shyness, feeling repressed.

If this chakra is over-active, there is a tendency towards being over emotional and being overly attached to people. This can generate feelings of constant drama, rocky relationships, accelerated lust.

Muladhara

~ Spiritual Message
~ Life Issues
~ Muladhara and the Glands
~ Muladhara, the Aura, and the Soul
~ An Out of Balance Muladhara

Muladhara, pronounced: *mool-ard-ara*, and is Sanskrit for root or support.

Generically it is known as the base or root chakra, and is symbolized by a lotus with four petals and associated with the color red.

Its spiritual function is physical survival, instincts, security, survival and also to basic human potentiality. The Kundalini lies coiled here, ready to uncoil and bring man to his highest spiritual potential in the crown chakra. The dormant power of the Kundalini rests within this chakra. The Kundalini is a great mystery; however, it represents a transformative force of awakening. The complete rising of this force brings liberation and enlightenment and as it rises up through the chakras it transforms all in its path. There is a particular polarity between this chakra and that of the crown. The base chakra holds the root of the Kundalini; the crown chakra opens fully at the time of `flowering'.

Located at the base of the spine near the coccyx (tail-bone) and although no endocrine organ is placed here, it is linked to the gonads, the adrenal medulla, responsible for the 'flight or fight' response when survival is under threat.

Spiritual Message
Physical functioning and sensation, and being connected to the earth plane through being center.

Life Issues

The life issues associated with this chakra involve physical family and group safety and security, ability to provide for life's necessities and stand up for oneself, feeling at home, social and familial law and order, abandonment fears, family bonding, identity, tribal honor code, support and loyalty.

Muladhara's sacred truth is all is one — we are connected to all of life. Every choice we make and every belief we hold exerts influence upon the whole of life.

Muladhara and the Glands

The Muladhara chakra is associated with the reproductive glands. It is the center of physical energy, grounding and self-preservation. Also governing the adrenals and represents the physical will-to-be, providing the extra energy to deal with stress and overcome obstacles.

Muladhara, the Aura, and the Soul

Muladhara correlates with the area of consciousness of the physical body and all physical sensations, including, pleasure, pain, as well as rage emanates from this center. Every chakra affects and is affected by the physical body and its health and functioning. Every chakra, except the Muladhara, also connects to a 'subtle body'. This chakra, with its lowest vibration rate, is the chakra of matter and is linked to the most solid aspects of the physical body.

Through acceptance of incarnation, we become 'rooted' into the element of earth and life of the planet. This is part of the grounding process that esoteric teaching espouses; when we are grounded we find peace. The more we are grounded, the less burden life on earth becomes. Difficulties take on a new perspective, giving us more over-all purpose and a sense of meaning.

A sense of feeling grounded becomes the foundation for the

development of the fullest potential possible in each individual. Strengthening this chakra re-balances instinctual judgment and when balanced it is positively active bringing a sense of purpose, belonging to the natural world and a willingness to take personal responsibility for actions and deeds.

The Muladhara chakra is a powerful anchor which links us with all living things. It is our base in the physical world. A sense of belonging to the physical world is vital in our dealings with it. If we believe ourselves to be separate from the natural world as outsiders, observers and manipulators we make a grave error. This chakra is about the will to survive and without this there is no willingness to battle against adverse circumstances or to adapt to new situations. This chakra, unlike the others faces downwards towards the earth where it picks up and transmits subtle forces.

An Out of Balance Muladhara

Possible physical areas affected by an out of balance chakra:
Anorexia, obesity, osteoarthritis, auto-immune disease, arthritis, cancer, aids, fatigue, kidney, spinal column, chronic lower back pain, rectal and immune disorders, depression, multiple personality disorder, obsessive-compulsive disorder, addictions, sciatica, varicose veins.

Possible spiritual/emotional areas affected by an out of balance chakra:
The Root chakra is about being physically 'there' and feeling at home and 'grounded' in situations. Its function is physical survival, instincts, security, survival and also to basic human potentiality. If it is open, we will feel grounded, stable and secure in a sense of feeling 'present' in the 'here and now' and connected to our physical body.

When under-active there is a tendency towards fearful or nervousness and this can generate feelings of fear of death, fear of change, stress, insecurity, lack of grounded-ness, need to shop or hoard to feel safe.

When over-active there is a tendency towards being material-istic, obstinate and greedy along with the possibility of feeling obsessed with security and resisting change. This can generate feelings of feelings of aggression, impulsive and reckless actions.

Chakra Imbalance Test

Here is a simple test you can do yourself to identify imbalances in the chakras. It is recommended that you seek a professional practitioner if in doubt or for regular balancing. The self testing process is performed via a body barometer test or otherwise known as an *ideokinetic test*. The term *ideokinetic* relates to an idea or thought connecting with a motor or muscular response. An ideokinetic energy test demonstrates exactly that, even if the idea/thought is subconscious rather than conscious.

Using the ideokinetic test will involve using the entire body, standing upright. Using the analogy of a tree learning towards the sun, the human body inclines naturally toward what agrees with it.

Try it now. Stand and ensure your feet are hip measurement apart and firmly on the floor with hands to the side. Think 'yes', with a strong positive feeling. Wait, and notice your body's subtle response to 'yes'. It will naturally sway slightly forward. Repeat this a few times for practice. Now think 'no', and notice your body's response to 'no'. It will lean slightly back or to the side.

Ideokinetic Test

1. Mentally set the intention that a balanced chakra is 'yes' and a sway forward and an imbalance in the chakra is 'no' and a sway backward.

2. Take a deep breath and close your eyes. Hold both hands, (one hand on top of the other), over the crown chakra — top of head. Leave your hands there until your body sways forward or backwards. Once you have received your indicator either 'yes' or 'no' take note of it.

3. You are ready to move on to the next chakra — the third

eye chakra, again placing both hands on the area between your eyebrows or brow area. Once you have your indicator either 'yes' or 'no' take note of it.

4. Continue this process through the rest of the chakras:

5. **Throat Chakra** — place both hands on the area of the adams apple

6. **Thymus Chakra** — place both hands on the area just above the breast bone

7. **Solar Plexus Chakra** — on the navel area

8. **Sacral Chakra** — place both hands on the area just below the navel and above the pubic bone

9. **Base Chakra** — place both hands over the pubis area

10. Once completed look at your notations and you should be able to identify the out of balance chakras.

11. The next step involves balancing the chakras one-by-one. As chakras work in harmony with each other there will always be another chakra to act as a balancer.

12. Always balance chakras top to bottom, i.e. from crown to base chakras. Start with the first chakra identified and place right hand over the area. In the next step we are going to identify which chakra will balance this one. Moving to the base chakra place your left hand and wait for your sway indicator. For example, let's assume you are working with the third eye chakra. Place your right hand on the brow area and the left hand on the base chakra, if

the sway reveals 'no', move to the sacral chakra and continue moving through the chakras until you get a 'yes' response. The 'yes' response is the one you need to balance the chakra. Once identified, hold your right hand over the area of the out of balance chakra and your left hand on the balancing chakra until you receive an indicator; this can come as a deep breath or a sway response of a 'yes'.

13. Continue through all of the out-of-balance chakras one by one as illustrated in step 7 until you have balanced and aligned your chakra system. You can re-test the out of balance chakras if you desire simply by placing both hands on the out of balance chakra identified in step 5 — if your body sways 'yes' you have successfully corrected the imbalance.

14. NB each chakra can have different support balancers.

15. Final step is to look back on the endocrine gland and the meridian linked to the chakra that was 'out-of-balance'. Continue support of this chakra with supports for meridian and endocrine.

Table 3 Chakra and Meridian Correlations

Meridian	Element	Chakra Primary	Chakra Secondary
Stomach Meridian	Earth	Solar Plexus *Manipura*	Throat *Vishuddha* Heart Anahata Brow *Ajna*
Spleen Meridian	Earth	Sacral *Svadhisthana*	Heart *Anahata*
Heart Meridian	Fire	Heart *Anahata*	
Small Intestine Meridian	Fire	Sacral *Svadhisthana*	Throat *Vishuddha*
Bladder Meridian	Water	Base *Muladhara*	Brow *Ajna* Crown *Sahasrara*
Kidney Meridian	Water	Base *Muladhara*	Throat *Vishuddha* Heart Anahata Solar Plexus *Manipura* Sacral *Svadhisthana*
Circulation Sex Meridian	Fire	Sacral *Svadhisthana*	Heart *Anahata*
Triple Warmer	Fire	Brow *Ajna*	Throat *Vishuddha*

Meridian

Gall Bladder Meridian	**Wood**	Solar Plexus *Manipura*	Crown *Sahasrara*
Liver Meridian	**Wood**	Solar Plexus *Manipura*	Base *Muladhara*
Lung Meridian	**Metal**	Heart Anahata	
Large Intestine Meridian	**Metal**	Solar Plexus *Manipura*	Throat *Vishuddha*
Central Meridian		Throat *Vishuddha* Heart Anahata Base *Muladhara* Solar Plexus *Manipura* Sacral *Svadhisthana*	
Governing Meridian		Base *Muladhara* Brow *Ajna* Crown *Sahasrara*	

PART THREE:
PUTTING IT ALL TOGETHER

Live in rooms full of light
Avoid heavy food
Be moderate in the drinking of wine
Take massage, baths, exercise, and gymnastics
Fight insomnia with gentle rocking or the sound of running water
Change surroundings and take long journeys
Strictly avoid frightening ideas
Indulge in cheerful conversation and amusements
Listen to music.

~ A Cornelius Celsus ~

Putting It All Together

The healing process and sustaining health involves a plan and a way of putting the information together. In a fast-paced world, it is easy to overwork, take on too many commitments, and extend to the point of exhaustion. Finding time to support and nourish our bodies can become just another task. This section demonstrates a plan and a way to incorporate simple techniques into daily regimes with minimal disruption or the need to find extra time in the day. If we take care of ourselves by eating properly, getting enough rest, implementing simple exercises, and practicing techniques that release tension and balance our bodies — then our *Personal Tuning Fork* has an opportunity to do its job.

Identifying Pain or Discomfort

Most people experience pain or discomfort. If this is your reason for reading this book, then before we begin I encourage you to begin here and follow these simple steps.

1. Many factors interfere with optimum functioning of the endocrine system. When the delicate hormonal balance is maintained our body performs many vital functions. Because the endocrine system is so complex and carefully calibrated, a variety of problems can result due to an imbalance. Glance through the tables of imbalance and take note of any symptoms you identify with. Re-read the chapter on that particular gland and always see your medical professional for assistance and correct diagnosis.

An imbalance anywhere in the endocrine system results in general lack of wellbeing demonstrated in:

Anxiety or depression	Loss of libido	Hair loss
Allergies	Low basal temperature (below 97.8)	Headaches
Appetite changes	Low tolerance for pain	Weight loss or gain
Back pain	Memory lapses	Yeast infections
Blood Pressure low or high	Menstrual irregularities	Puffiness of the throat or face
Brittle hair and nails	Mood swings	Sugar cravings
Bruising easily	Muscular cramps or twitching	Sweating
Chemical sensitivities	Poor circulation	Swollen glands
Cold hands and feet	Poor memory or concentration	Excessive urination/fluid imbalance
Constipation	Poor nutrient assimilation	Fatigue/insomnia
Digestive problems	Lowered immune	Dry or itchy skin
Dizziness	Diarrhea	Sleep disorders

2. In this next step I suggest you grade your pain or discomfort. By doing this you will have a gauge by which you can measure progress.

Visualize your pain or discomfort or general lack of wellbeing along a horizontal line with 0 at the left end, minimal or no pain and 10 at the right end, maximum pain.

(You can be more specific if you want and use for example fatigue, lowered immunity, irritability, foggy thinking, depression or any other ailment you currently experience).

0 _____ 10

Mark where you are on this scale and date it.

Now draw up another scale and place a realistic mark where you would like it to be in say, a week's time.

It is always good to visualize where you want to be and what that means to you. It is about recognizing yourself holistically. By engaging the imagination and giving yourself a goal to work towards, the subconscious begins the process — it is almost as if the subconscious says '*Yes! we are on the way to wellbeing!*', thus the healing process commences. Simply engaging the mind with the physical brings cohesion and you are on the way to achieving your desired outcome.

Using a visual analogue scale on a piece of paper you can record your daily or weekly progress with colored markers.

Fatigue and low energy
0 _____| 10

Where I would like to be
0 _____| 10

Now mark down what changes you may have to make to ensure

the desired outcome. For example, it could be supporting yourself more with nutrition and time out to walk on the beach every day with a spot of mediation whilst you are at the beach. It could be seeking out the reflexologist and drinking more water or working with the chakras and meridian points combined with balancing your thoughts about your partner, work or financial situation.

Trust your subconscious during this process and attempt to select the processes that you are comfortable with whilst challenging your comfort zones.

Longevity, youthfulness, health and beauty depend upon the optimum functioning of the endocrine system. The glands and the hormones secreted are vital to rejuvenation of the body and once they begin to deteriorate, aging and ill-health occur.

The healing process is one of softening, opening up and letting go. It manifests when the vital force increases and body fluids and pressures are equalized, thus facilitating the communication of function on all levels, including the subtle body to the physical body.

A Healthy Plan

As a healing process can generate the elimination of negative, toxic, destructive and unassimilated residues on all levels, supporting this process with a healthy plan assists the fragile nature of restoration.

Health is a dynamic process of being in the present and allowing life to flow in and out at all levels. Areas of stress, congestion, or depletion are relieved and balanced to make way for positive, cleansing and regenerative forces.

Thus, the healing process involves a healthy plan. A supported healthy plan and treatment precipitates a release of positivity needed to overthrow accumulated resistant negativity, whether this is habit, thoughts, emotions, nutrient, inertia, stress, tears, laughter ... this can be and is often different for everyone.

Whatever treatment you embark upon it is helpful to ask the following questions and to consider the physical, emotional, mental and spiritual aspects of the problem.

- What am I taking into myself that is good for me?

- What am I taking into myself that is not good for me?

- What is the balance between what I am taking in and what I am eliminating?

- What am I eliminating that is good and what am I eliminating that is not?

- What am I holding on to that is good?

- What am I holding on to that is not good?

- How am I stopping the elimination of what is not good for me?

- What can I do to let go of what is harmful to me?

- How can I increase my acceptance of what is good for me?

The above questions will help you to take a clear look at that is happening in your life. Once you can see what you have to do, it is only a matter of time until it is achieved. Conscious recognition and acceptance is the first step. You are now on your way towards total wellbeing via a balanced and healthy Personal Tuning Fork — holistically — homeostatically.

As part of a healthy plan for healthy living it is necessary to engage in healthy approaches. The following guide can assist you in making healthy choices.

Therapies for a Healthy Endocrine

"Health is not valued until sickness comes."
~ Thomas Fuller ~

Today it seems, particularly in western culture, any health modality that does not fit the conventional-medicine-practices, falls into the category of alternative medicine. Hence, there is a degree of skepticism, mystery and even a little dismissive poopooing that goes on when the subject of alternative practices or complimentary therapies arises.

Yet, in Eastern and indigenous cultures the practice of such alternatives for healing are standard practice. One could question *who is right?* Both have there place. In defense of alternative practices (assuming they need defense) they do focus on individualizing treatments, good nutrition and preventive practices, balanced lifestyle, treating the whole person, promoting self-care and self-healing, understanding the connection between the physical form and the subtle energies and recognizing the spiritual nature of each individual.

The past decade has seen tremendous growth in alternative medicine techniques. There are more practitioners, more modalities, there is more information, more research and greater accessibility ...

At the end of the day, it is about finding what works for you, being open to alternative practices and applying them as a complementary to traditional medicine. Holistic, naturopathic, alternative or complementary therapies are a wonderful way to support and restore health. They work on the body in its entirety towards balancing the body's energetic system to restore homeostasis. Some therapies target more specific systems, most have a domino effect upon the body's state of well-being.

There are numerous therapies one could use:

Acupuncture
Fine needles are inserted at specific points to stimulate, disperse, and regulate the flow of vital energy, and restore a healthy energy balance. Acupuncture has a general tonifying effect on the whole endocrine system to improve physical health, treat hormonal imbalances, ease anxiety or offer pain relief.

Acupressure
Similar to acupuncture, but using finger pressure rather than fine needles on specific points along the body to treat ailments such as tension and stress, aches and pains, menstrual cramps, arthritis.

Read more about acupressure in the chapter 'Acupressure Points and the Endocrine'.

Aromatherapy
Using essential oils distilled from plants, aromatherapy treats emotional disorders such as headaches, stress and anxiety. Essential oils are similar to the body's chemical messengers so aromatherapy can ease hormonally influenced ailments such as premenstrual disorders. Oils are massaged into the skin in diluted form, inhaled, or placed in baths.

Ayurvedic Medicine
Practiced in India for more than 5,000 years; ayurvedic tradition holds that illness is a state of imbalance among the body's systems that can be detected through diagnostic procedures such as reading the pulse and observing the tongue. Can treat phlegm, balance blood pressure, and improve energy levels.

Bach Flower Remedies
A system of herbal remedies devised by Edward Bach; these

floral remedies alter the disharmonies of personality and emotional state that trouble us all from time to time.

Read more about these amazing home remedies in the chapter 'Bach Flower Remedies'.

Color Therapy
The use of colored light shone onto the pineal gland and other important points on the endocrine system to produce beneficial or healing effects in all dimensions of time.

See more about this unique therapy in the chapter 'Color Therapies'.

Counseling/Psychotherapy
It is about freeing up the emotions in connection with physical symptoms. Addresses, depression, stress, self esteem issues, addiction, and grief, exploring the underlying issues or focusing on coping mechanisms, depending on the type of psychotherapy.

Read more about the emotions and thoughts in the chapters 'Thoughts and Emotions' and 'Emotional Counseling'.

Crystal Therapy
A relatively recent discovery in the field of alternative medicines, it involves the use of specific gem stones to rebalance the flow of energy in the auric field and sometimes allowing the mineral content of the gems to help restore health .

Herbalism
Herbal medicine is an ancient form of healing that is still widely used. Herbalism uses the leaves, stems, roots or seeds of naturally growing plants to treat a range of illness symptoms, from high fever or digestive upsets to wound healing, and mental imbalances such as stress, anxiety and insomnia.. Many modern pharmaceutical medications from cancer drugs to

aspirin are based on research into medicinal effects of chemicals naturally occurring in plants (such as willow bark).

Read more about the use of herbs for healing in the chapter 'Herbs and Foods for Healthy Endocrine'.

Homoeopathy

A medical system that uses infinitesimal doses of natural mineral plant or animal substances to stimulate a person's immune and defense system. The right remedy individually selected for a person's whole state of mind and physical symptoms can re-harmonize mental and emotional wellbeing, heal the symptoms in acute or chronic conditions and cure the underlying susceptibility to recurring ailments.

Read more about the homeopathy in the chapter 'Schuessler Cell Salts'.

Iridology

A diagnostic system based on the premise that every organ has a corresponding location within the iris of the eye, which can serve as an indicator of the individual organ's health or disease.

Kinesiology

Kinesiology is the study of the human body during movement. There are many disciplines within Kinesiology including anatomy, biomechanics, exercise physiology, motor control, motor learning, neuromuscular physiology, sports psychology, and philosophy. It is commonly used for diagnosing the body's sensitivities or food intolerances.

Massage

The practice of manipulating a person's muscles and other soft tissue with moves such as effleurage, deep tissue, percussion, vibration, and joint movement, for improving a person's circulation, lymphatic drainage, unraveling knots of stress held in the muscles, promoting relaxation, health and well-being.

Meditation

By selecting a quiet place free from noise and distraction, sitting or resting quietly with eyes closed (usually on a floor), and trying to achieve a feeling of peace through meditation. There are various types of meditation - TM (Transcendental Meditation), mindfulness meditation, and from the Eastern tradition, Zen meditation, Buddhist meditation, and Taoist meditation.

Read more about meditation in the chapters 'Care of the Soul' and 'Breathing Techniques'.

Naturopathic Medicine

Naturopathic physicians work to restore and support the body's own healing abilities using a variety of modalities including nutrition, herbal medicine, homeopathic medicine, and oriental medicine.

Reflexology

Based on the idea that specific points on the feet and hands correspond with organs and tissues throughout the body. With fingers and thumbs, the practitioner applies pressure to these points to treat a wide range of stress-related illnesses.

Refer to the 'feet tapping points' image in the chapter 'Acupressure Points and the Endocrine'.

Reiki

Practitioners of this ancient Tibetan healing system use light hand placements to channel healing energies to the recipient.

Sound Therapy

Otherwise known as Sound Wave Energy healing, this is a holistic approach to healing the physical, mental, emotional, and spiritual aspects of the person through the use of sound frequencies. The focus is on returning the individual to a state of harmony and balance.

Therapeutic Touch

A non-invasive, holistic approach to healing based on principles of an energy exchange between people - sensing the aura around the body. It is about rebalancing the energy field by directing the flow thereby removing any blockages.

For more information regarding the aura and balancing techniques refer to the chapter in part two on the subtle body systems, 'The Aura'.

Yoga Therapy

The use of yoga asana positions and breathing to address mental and physical problems integrating mind, body and spirit.

Yoga is especially beneficial for the respiratory, circulatory, muscular, skeletal, immune and endocrine systems in particular the pituitary and thyroid glands. It lowers blood sugar levels and blood pressure, calms the mind and relaxes the body's core vital systems.

Read more about the practice of yoga in the chapter 'Yoga for the Endocrine'.

High on Acid

"My inner advisor is dying to heal me."
~ Astrid Alauda ~

Foods can be either acid forming, balancing or alkaline forming according to the condition they create in the body after being eaten. PH stands for potential of hydrogen or the amount of hydrogen molecules (positively charged molecules). A pH of 7.0 is neutral, below 7 is acidic and above 7 is alkaline.

For example:

0_____Vinegar_____7 Water_____Baking soda ___14

It is much easier to maintain a healthy pH than to try to regain balance after becoming acidic. For good health we need to keep our blood within a narrow pH range of around 6.5 to 7.3 if this is not evident, the body will seek out ways to help preserve this. For example, if your blood pH is too acidic, the body will seek out alkaline minerals like calcium and potassium to help buffer the excess acidity. If these minerals are not available, the body borrows them from the bones, tissues and organs. When tissues are robbed of minerals, it can cause bone spurs, osteoporosis, fatigue, heart palpitations, kidney stones and many other problems. If the acid load is too much for the blood to deal with, excess acid is dumped into the body's tissues for storage. The lymph and immune system try to neutralize this which means dumping it back into the blood and leaching out more minerals thereby stressing the major organs and impairing the endocrine system.

Symptoms Associated with Increased Acid Formation

Beginning Symptoms of Acidosis

Acne, endocrine disturbances, agitation, anxiety, diarrhea, dilated pupils, extraverted behavior, fatigue in early morning, headaches, hyperactivity, hyper sexuality, insomnia, nervousness, rapid heartbeat, restless legs, shortness of breath, strong appetite, high blood pressure, warm dry hands, muscular pain, cold hands and feet, dizziness, low energy, joint pains, food allergies, chemical sensitivity, panic attacks, pre-menstrual and menstrual cramping, anxiety and depression, lack of sex drive, bloating, heartburn, constipation, strong smelling urine, irregular heartbeat, white coated tongue, excess head mucus, metallic taste in mouth.

Intermediate Symptoms of Acidosis

Endocrine disturbances, Herpes I & 11, depression, loss of memory, loss of consciousness, migraine, headaches, insomnia, disturbances in smell, taste, vision, hearing, asthma, hay fever, earaches, hives, swelling, viral infections, bacterial infections (staph, strep), fungal infections, impotence, cystitis, urinary track infections, gastritis, colitis, excessive hair loss, psoriasis, endometriosis, diarrhea, stuttering, numbness & tingling and sinusitis.

Advanced Symptoms of Acidosis

Endocrine breakdown, Crohn's disease, schizophrenia, learning disabilities, Hodgkin's disease, lupus, multiple sclerosis, osteoporosis, rheumatoid and osteo arthritis, leukemia, tuberculosis and cancer.

Generating Balance

Every cell within the human body and every metabolic process depends on the right pH balance. This includes the endocrine system. The best way to restore balance is to return the body back towards an alkaline and oxygenated state.

So how do you know if you are too acidic? Firstly, you should know by the way you feel and any symptoms you are exhibiting. Secondly, you can check your pH with pH strips. It is best to test the pH of your urine as the pH of saliva changes too much throughout the day. The strips will change color according to your pH. This will help you to identify trends in your pH according to what you are eating.

How do you correct this imbalance and your internal environment? The only way to return the correct pH to your blood is by taking steps to re-alkalize your system. The best way to generate balance is through dietary steps — eating a diet comprising 80% alkaline-forming foods and 20% acid-forming foods.

Acid/Alkaline Foods

Western diets are rich in acid-forming processed foods, red meats, refined grains and sugar and very low in alkaline-forming foods like fresh fruits and vegetables. An ideal diet should be 80% alkaline and 20% acidic.

Alkaline-Forming Foods, Substances

Alkaline-Forming Vegetables
Alfalfa, asparagus, artichoke, avocado, barley grass, beet greens, beetroot, broccoli, brussel sprout, burdock, cabbage, capsicum (red, yellow, green), carrots, cauliflower, celery, chard, chicory, chives, chlorella, collard, cucumber, daikon, dandelion, endive, fennel, garlic, ginger, green and yellow squash, green bean, kale, kamut grass, leek, lettuce, mushrooms, mustard greens, nightshade vegetables, okra, onion, parsley, parsnip, pea, pumpkin, radish, reishi, seaweed and sea vegetable (nori, wakame, hijike),

shitake, spinach, spring onion, sprouted grains, beans and seeds, swiss chard, sweet potato, sprouts, spirulina, taro, turnip, wasabi, water chestnut, watercress, winter squash and wheat-grass.

Alkaline-Forming Fruits

Apple, apricot, avocado, blackcurrant, banana, berries, blueberry, cantaloupe, cherry, coconut, currant, date, fig, grape, grapefruit, honeydew melon, kiwi, lemon, lime, mandarin, mango, melon, nectarine, orange, papaya, peach, pear, pineapple, raisin, raspberry, strawberry, tangerine, tomato, tropical fruits, umeboshi plum, watermelon.

Alkaline-Forming Protein

Hemp protein, millet, tempeh and tofu, organic soy milk, soy cheese, soy lecithin, soured dairy products.

Alkaline-Forming Grains and Legumes

Non-stored organic grains like millet, buckwheat, quinoa, amaranth, any sprouted grain or legume, black-eyed peas.

Alkaline Seeds and Nuts

Almond, sesame seed, almond milk, brazil nut, caraway, chia seed, flaxseed, hazelnut, chestnut, poppy seed, pumpkin seed.

Alkaline-Forming Sweeteners, Condiments, Spices, Oils

Apple cider vinegar, stevia, cinnamon, curry, ginger, mustard, cayenne, chilli pepper, sea salt, miso, tamari and all herbs, olive oil, flaxseed oil, evening primrose oil, marine lipids, borage oil, blackstrap molasses, brown rice vinegar.

Other Alkalizing Substances

Bee pollen, lecithin granules, probiotic cultures, green juices, soured dairy products, vegetable juices, mineral water, green tea, herbal tea, raw goat milk, agar agar, positive emotions, alkaline energized water at pH of 8 and above.

Alkaline Minerals
Cesium, potassium, sodium, calcium and magnesium.

Acid-Forming Foods, Substances

Acid-Forming Vegetables
Corn, olives, winter squash, any tinned vegetables.

Acid-Forming Fruits
Blackberry, canned or glazed fruit, cranberry, plum, prune.

Acid-Forming Grains, Beans and Legumes
Barley, bran (wheat), bran (oat), chickpea, corn, cornstarch, kamut, lentil, oat (rolled), oatmeal, pinto bean, red bean, white bean, white rice, rye, spelt, wheat, wheat germ, noodle, macaroni, spaghetti, bread, crackers, white flour, wheat flour.

Acid-Forming Dairy
Cheese, ice cream, milk (homogenised and pasteurised), egg.

Acid-Forming Nuts and Seeds
Cashew, peanut, peanut butter, pecan, tahini, walnut, pistachio.

Acid-Forming Protein
Bacon, beef, chicken, carp, clams, cod, corned beef, fish, haddock, lamb, lobster, mussels, organ meats, oysters, pike, pork, rabbit, salmon, sardines, sausage, scallops, shrimp, shellfish, tuna, turkey, veal, venison.

Acid-Forming Sweeteners, Condiments, Oils
Canola oil, carob, corn syrup, cocoa, vinegar, mustard, pepper,

sugar in any form including white, brown or cane sugar, maple syrup, honey (mild), sucrose, fructose, maltose, lactose, glucose, sorbitol, sesame, corn and sunflower oil, chocolate, gelatine, mayonnaise, jam, jelly, MSG, table salt, vinegar.

Acid-Forming Beverages
Beer, spirits, hard liquor, wine, soft drink, coffee, most tap water.

Other Acid-Forming Substances
Aspirin, chemicals, drugs, pesticides, herbicides, tobacco, any processed or junk food, stress, worry, anger and negative emotions.

Neutral Foods
Butter (fresh), cream (raw, fresh), cow's milk and whey (raw and fresh), vegetable oils (unprocessed), yoghurt (acidophilus, raw), fresh coconut meat, xylitol and ghee.

Stress

"It is not the events of your life that cause stress, but the way you think about them."
"Man (sic) is not disturbed by things but by the views he takes of them."
~ Epictetus, 120 AD ~

There is so much information available today regarding stress in relation to wellbeing. So much so that it would be difficult to ignore the effects of stress upon our health, much less how we can manage stress. Yet, it can be difficult often times to be aware of our stress levels as we conduct our day to day lives.

Yes, stress can be a factor in disease and often it is the bringer of inner chaos born out of outer chaos. Stress has the power to prohibit recovery, throw out equilibrium and affect our wellbeing aggressively compromising sustainable health.

As a contributing factor towards ill-health, stress demands discussion.

Stress has its own modus operandi and performs like a reactive event or trigger — creating the *stress cycle*.

The Stress Cycle or 'Flight or Fight' Reaction

Stage 1 - Thoughts
Stress begins with your thoughts. Problematic stress occurs when you think negatively about whatever is stressing you. For example, you could be stressed regarding a particular health issue, couple that stress with thoughts of negativity such as — *I will never be well again ... I hate this situation ... no one supports me* and so on.

Stage 2 - Emotions
Negative thoughts produce negative emotions. A thought generated in the cortex of the brain is triggered in the mid brain as an emotion consistent or comparable with the thought, be it fear, anger, guilt, hatred, anxiety, regret, remorse, grief, sadness, jealousy, embarrassment or any other negative emotion.

Stage 3 - Chemical Reactions
This involves the sympathetic nervous system and the endocrine or hormonal system. The negative thought sends nerve impulses to the adrenal glands, which release a number of different chemicals into the blood stream. These circulate via the blood stream throughout the body, affecting the pituitary gland, where it releases more chemicals. These are known as stress chemicals and include corticosteroids such as adrenaline and noradrenaline, other hormones and neuro-transmitters.

Stage 4 - Physical Symptoms of Stress
The stress chemicals activate every organ in the body. Their physical effects are most noticeable when the emotion is intense. These physical symptoms of stress include:

- Heart - Increased heart rate, irregular breathing, palpitations.

- Stomach - Increased secretion of hydrochloric acid into the stomach, butterflies, burning, churning, nausea, vomiting.

- Gut - Increased stomach pains, diarrhea, increased frequency of urination.

- Muscles - Muscle constriction, headaches, stiff necks, sore backs, chest tightness, twitching.

- Lungs - Constriction of lungs and bronchial tubes, breathing irregularities, sighing, yawning, hyperventilation.

- Tear Glands - Tearfulness.

- Sweat Glands - Increased sweating.

- Salivary Glands - Decreased saliva, dry mouth or throat.

- Skin - Increased blood flow to the skin resulting in flushing, red rash and temperature increase. With prolonged stress, blood flow increase to central body core resulting in feelings of coldness, pins and needles.

- Brain - Dilation of cranial arteries resulting in migraine, sleep problems and interference with the brain's neuro-transmitters which results in stage fright, memory and concentration problems, difficulty making decisions, dizziness and fainting.

- Immune System - Destruction of leukocytes or white blood cells, increasing vulnerability to disease.

As the stress chemicals pass through the brain they set off further negative thoughts and so perpetuate the cycle. Once stress starts, it is likely to continue. Long-term stress can cause or exacerbate many physical ailments. These include heart attacks, asthma, ulcers, irritable bowel, colitis, spots, eczema, dermatitis, alopecia (hair loss), dandruff, herpes, shingles, high blood pressure, strokes, and such immune related illnesses as colds, pneumonia, bronchitis and influenza. According to some researchers, diabetes, multiple sclerosis, auto-immune disorders,

AIDS and cancer are all more likely with prolonged stress.

Non-physical ailments due to stress include personality problems such as increased pessimism, increased irritability/ anger, and loss of confidence. Phobias, depression, burn-out, panic attacks, schizophrenic and manic-depressive episodes can also be triggered by stress.

The only effective long-term strategies are those which shut off the cycle at stage one, i.e. those that prevent the flow on effect of negative thinking. The adrenals and pineal gland are especially affected by stress and the stress cycle. In all, stress inhibits hormone flow throughout the endocrine system.

Supportive measures for stress include, meditation, affir-mation, visualization, leisure pursuits, changes in thought processes including those around the stressor, changes in lifestyle, laughter and some would say chocolate. Being aware of the stress cycle enables a state of control over the cycle particu-larly when placing an intervention at a point of significance in the cycle process. The same applies to an awareness with regard to your own stress cycle and how you manifest stress in your habits, thoughts, physical symptoms and behaviors.

Nutrition

"If I'd known I was going to live so long, I'd have taken better care of myself."
~ **Leon Eldred** ~

Hormones react very sensitively to things we eat and some endocrine disorders are related to diet and nutrition. So the single most effective preventive measure is to eat nutritious, healthy meals, minimize alcohol consumption and avoid tobacco and drugs. Our body's organs and the endocrine system do not respond well to foods high in sugar, fats or highly processed refined foods.

Nutrition is vital in building resistance to illness. Processed foods have been stripped of necessary nutrients and fiber. This renders them to a devitalized state and consuming them weakens the immune system decreasing resistance to disease. Certain foods, such as miso soup, parsley, beans, tofu, sea vegetables, fresh vegetables, and lightly toasted sesame seeds can strengthen the immune system reinforcing the body's ability to protect itself.

Foods to be avoided are mucous forming foods such as dairy, sugar, white flour products and processed foods.

It is possible to improve thymus function through consuming seaweed products, spirulina, soy protein, organic fruits and vegetables, grains, nuts and seeds.

Minerals and herbs play an important role and they assist by feeding the endocrine system and specific glands.

When re-assessing nutrition it is important to consider how we eat. Rushing our food on the way to work, eating in front of the television or whilst having an argument or when stressed will affect assimilation of minerals and vitamins impairing digestion.

Environment

"Health is a large word. It embraces not the body only, but the mind and spirit as well... and not today's pain or pleasure alone, but the whole being and outlook of a man."
~ *James H. West* ~

Whilst it is difficult to avoid some day-to-day environmental factors, ensuring your environment is conducive towards total wellbeing is paramount. For example, if you are required to spend lengthy periods behind the computer, take frequent breaks and walk in the fresh air and sunshine. Avoid over-use of chemicals and exposure to chemically charged activities or environments such as cleaning materials, fuel and smoking.

Another environmental factor can be the people around you in your day to day life or at work. Unfortunately at an endocrinal level, people can affect us more than we may think. What does this mean? Should we place consideration upon our choice of friends, associates, husbands, wives, family members? Naturally, this is neither practical nor desirable when considering family and loved ones. However, we can raise our 'life energy' when in the presence of those who affect our equilibrium adversely.

When our personal energies are strong, we are less likely to take on other's energies. In this way, our equilibrium will remain uncompromised when stressed or when in the company of stressful, upsetting people.

We can maintain our energy level through focus, being mindful of our own issues, awareness of what buttons are being pushed with regard to our own personal development, not taking what is said or done personally, managing our reactions or responses, cleansing our aura, monitoring thoughts, deflecting, asking questions, detachment with empathy, love, forgiveness, acceptance when we do not understand and remembering to breathe.

When considering other groups of people who we can dispense with — we should do just that — if they do not enhance our lives they most certainly will not enhance our health. We can dispense or avoid these people and situations.

Weight

"He who takes medicine and neglects to diet wastes the skill of his doctors."
~ Chinese Proverb ~

Keeping your body at a healthy weight will greatly diminish the risk of developing endocrine and hormonal disorders. In particular, maintaining a healthy weight assists conditions such as type II Diabetes Mellitus. The hormone insulin stimulates cells and tissues into action whereby it uses energy generated by the food we eat. Obesity increases the body's resistance to the action of insulin and this can result in diabetes. It can also interrupt thyroid function, which perpetuates the obesity cycle.

It would be fair to mention here that being under-weight equally poses problems for the body and in particular the adrenals. In this instance, the adrenals work harder and the tendency to become prey to adrenal over-load is heightened. Crash dieting and weight loss fads play havoc with the delicate balance of the endocrine system. Yes, balanced applications for weight loss or gain is the *go* here — so nutrition, exercise and holistic approaches that ensure optimum balance are the goals.

Determining your correct weight is considered the optimum approach to weight management. Along with monitoring ones habits in relation to your weight and the management of.

Remember, managing weight should be a holistic lifestyle choice not an isolated lifestyle fad. Remember the mind, body, soul principle. Cultivating positive thoughts nurtures the emotions. When we feel good we eat what is good for our body.

Breathing

"Breath is the bridge which connects life to consciousness, which unites your body to your thoughts."
~ Thich Nhat Hanh ~

Life is breath. Breath is life. We can live a long time without food, a couple of days without drinking, but life without breath is measured in minutes. Something so essential deserves our attention. Breath is the most important of all the bodily functions. There is a right way and a wrong way to breathe. Children breathe deeply from their diaphragm. As we age, however, our breathing shifts to the chest and becomes shallow and rapid. Right now, you are probably shallow breathing.

Shallow breathing doesn't give the muscles and brain the amount of air necessary for a healthy lifestyle. Shallow breathing impedes the natural states of relaxation, feeling good, and detoxification.

Deep breathing on the other hand, generates a flow of endorphins which help us feel good. It opens up pathways in the body's systems enabling a steady and balanced hormone flow. Deep breathing restores equilibrium and increases the ability to gain sustainable health.

Deep Breathing Techniques

Relax, close your eyes and begin to breath as normal.

Inhale slowly into the lower lungs.
Expand the sides, back, and front of the lower ribs.

Once lower lungs are filled, inhale more air into the upper chest.

Exhale air from upper chest very slowly.
Keep lower lungs full.

Contract abdominal muscles to push all air out.
Exhale remaining air. Relax.

A Breathing Exercise for the Endocrine System

Breathing should be slow and rhythmic - from the belly - filling the lungs before exhaling. This has a three-pronged effect; again, it is the mind, body, soul principle. It calms the emotions and centers the mind as well as oxygenating and detoxifying our body's systems.

Through a slow, gradual, inhale, and exhale you revitalize and energize your entire being. During the breathing process, place the tip of the tongue on the roof of the mouth, continue to breathe in rhythmically, exhale slowly and feel your entire being relax as it opens to the lightness of air. Even the bones, organs, brain and heart respond to this lightness. Thoughts feel lighter, the emotions less heavy and the spirit alive. The exhale is your opportunity to let go of stale air, emotions or anything you have been holding onto. It is an opportunity for every atom of your being to release the burden of the mind, heart, and body.

Focus on breathing deeply for two more minutes. Gently control your respiratory system, making each breath grow longer and deeper than the last one. Breathe out any tension you feel restricting your lungs from moving fully and naturally. Feel your mind clear with each breath. Notice any resistance your mind creates by way of worries and judgments. Take several deep breaths and dissolve these barriers.

Breathe deeply and gently; remember, you are breathing in life itself.

Hold the breath at the top of the exhalation for a moment, feeling its fullness. Then exhale smoothly, letting your hands drift down into your lap, and relax, feeling the vitality of the breath circulate throughout your body.

A Simple Breathing Exercise

Breathe in this ratio:

- Inhale for one count
- Hold for four counts
- Exhale for two counts

For example, if you inhale for 4 seconds, you hold for 16 and exhale for 8. Do sets of 10 breaths, 3 times a day spread out through the day. While staying within your comfort zone, progressively increase your seconds count to develop greater lung capacity. This is a tremendously beneficial practice for your health.

Exercise

"Those who think they have not time for bodily exercise will sooner or later, have to find time for illness."
~ Edward Stanley ~

Exercise can be anything that has you moving, whether it is walking the dog to vacuuming the carpet to playing catch with the kids to the more regimented pursuits such as jogging, swimming and sports. Exercise promotes a state of general wellbeing and assists in defusing stress in the body as it releases endorphins, which act as mood elevators.

Movement keeps the endocrine system moving, hormones flowing and chemicals active. In this way, hormones along with their associated endocrine chemicals are able to eliminate stress chemicals from the bloodstream. Stress chemicals if allowed to build up in the system, produce the physical symptoms of stress and this perpetuates the stress cycle.

Hence, movement and exercise is imperative in preventing or halting this process thus reducing stress and restoring the body to a state of homeostasis.

Simple techniques such as walks, stretches, dancing, running with the kids or your pets all enhance the endocrine system and constitute a form of exercise. Effects of yoga on glands can help regulate hormonal production and aids in the cleansing of the glands, thus improving their function. Aerobic exercise assists in managing stress, as exercise burns stress in the muscles and by use of the cardiovascular system.

Exercise for Endocrine Balancing

Exercise stimulates the thymus and lymph systems maintaining a healthy immune system. The following exercises are highly beneficial:

- *Squats* — moving up and down out of a squatting position will stimulate the thymus and the flow of lymph fluids. Use the 'Ha' breath with each squat.

- *Woodchopper* — imagine you are holding a rod-like instrument high above the head with legs hip width distance. With a swift movement, bring the imaginary item and your arms down between your legs as you shift into a squatting stance with legs bent. Again use the 'ha' breath and apply the sound. Cut through negativity and emotions with each movement.

- *Drain the Arches* — lie down close to a wall. Place your butt flush against the wall and raise the legs up vertical to your body and flush with the wall. A Yogic posture is excellent for stimulating the thymus and draining and flushing the spinal column

- *Sacroiliac Drainage* — lying on back, lift bent legs up until the knees rest on the abdomen. Wrap arms around the legs pulling them in towards the abdomen. Hold and then let go suddenly. Do on both sides. Repeating five times on each side.

Weeping

"Tears are the safety valve of the heart when too much pressure is laid on it."
~ Albert Smith ~

Weeping, crying, bawling, teary and so on — all of them are under-rated, berated and stigmatized. Yet, weeping is one of the most powerful natural function of cleansing and releasing stress. Weeping is one of the easiest and fastest ways to release toxins, raise energy levels and defuse stress.

Emotional tears are a response which are unique to humans. All animals that live in air produce tears to lubricate their eyes. But it is only humans that possess the marvelous system that creates the act of weeping.

Biochemist William Frey spent 15 years as head of a research team studying tears. His scientific studies found that tears created from 'emotional crying' carry toxins not normally found in the tear created to simply moisten the eye. The research team compared the normal moisturizing tear with the tear caused by emotion and found that stressful tears contained far more toxic biological by-products in addition to ACTH hormone, which is associated with high blood pressure, heart problems, peptic ulcers and other physical conditions closely related to stress.

Weeping, they concluded, is an excretory process which removes toxic substances from the body that normally build up during emotional stress.

The simple act of weeping not only cleanses and detoxifies, it raises the body's energy levels, which assists people to feel better both physically and physiologically. Suppressing tears increases stress levels, and contributes to diseases aggravated by stress, such as high blood pressure, heart problems and peptic ulcers.

And so it is … weeping contributes not only to the health of the individual, but at a more lateral level, tears are an extremely effective method of communication, and can elicit sympathy much faster than any other means, thus deepening connections with others.

Laughter

"A good laugh and a long sleep are the best cures in the doctor's book."
~ Irish Proverb ~

Laughter is one of the easiest and fastest ways to release toxins, raise energy levels and decrease stress. The act of laughing is gaining more insight today and accepted as a therapy as demonstrated through laughing clubs.

There appears to be an assumption that we need something funny to laugh at. The contrary is true. Children laugh approximately 80 to 100 times per day. Children appreciate the relationship between humor and enjoying life. They will laugh at anything! If you ask them, "What's so funny," they may say something like, "nothing!"

By the time we reach adulthood, we laugh only 5-6 times per day. It is not so much that we have lost the ability to laugh or forgotten how to but we simply do not find the time to or are too stressed to find the humor in — *nothing*.

Some of the benefits of laughter are:

- Enhances T-cell production, which boosts the immune system

- Triggers the release of endorphins, the body's natural painkillers

- Releases toxins

- Provides for improved cardio-pulmonary function

- Lowers blood pressure

- Reduces stress hormones

- Increases muscle flexion

- Raises levels of disease-fighting proteins called Gamma-interferon and B-cells, which produce disease-destroying antibodies

- Produces a general sense of wellbeing

- Dissolves tension, stress, anxiety, irritation, anger, grief, and depression

- Lowers inhibitions

- Releases pent-up emotions generating a sense of wellbeing.

- Helps to integrate both hemispheres of the brain

Laughter has the ability to raise the vibrations and energy levels of humans and is becoming one of the most low maintenance, free, all rounder holistic balancers available for better health. Plus it is contagious – a healthy contagious!

Rest and Relax

"Don't underestimate the value of doing nothing, of just going along, listening to all the things you can't hear, and not bothering."
~ Pooh's Little Instruction Book, inspired by A.A. Milne ~

Also important in maintaining a healthy endocrine system and general wellbeing, is to keep a balance in life. That is to ensure your life has vacations, recreational activities, events and activities that give you joy, satisfaction and a sense of achievement, reward and relaxation. In particular simple relaxation techniques which promote stillness and quiet within the body such as breathing, meditation, silence — doing nothing.

There are a number of ways we can encourage our body to relax:

Stress de-activating buttons
Stress de-activating buttons is about engaging the 'Centering Button' and the 'Stress Release Button'.

- The 'Centering Button' is located at the roof of your mouth. The tip of the tongue is placed against the roof of the mouth, about a quarter of an inch behind the upper front teeth. This has the effect of what we call being centered or strengthened and assists in the relaxation process.

- The 'Stress Release Button' is located three finger widths below your navel. Locate this spot and apply pressure into the belly region. Hold for 30 seconds, remember to breathe. Release the pressure with an outward breath. This action releases stress from the adrenal glands.

Do What You Love to Do

Participate in a favorite activity such as going to the cinema, reading a book, listening to music, shopping. Anything that switches your mind towards something other than that which you normally engage in.

Do Nothing

Do nothing. This is a very difficult thing for many people. Doing nothing is quite under-valued and the power of doing nothing in terms of rejuvenating our bodies is grossly under-estimated. If you do find it difficult to do nothing, begin with small increments, even if it is for ten minutes and slowly build up until you can successfully do nothing for a minimum of one hour per day.

Laugh and Sing

Singing and laughing, even the simple act of smiling assists in the relaxation process. These actions and movements relax the facial muscles and the muscles surrounding the cranium. Studies have revealed that these functions also assist in lowering the heart rate and engages full breathing into the diaphragm and belly.

Education and Tuning Within

"In minds crammed with thoughts, organs clogged with toxins, and bodies stiffened with neglect, there is just no space for anything else."
~ Alison Rose Levy ~

Education

Knowing your family medical history is important to your health. Among the familial endocrine disorders are diabetes and hypothyroidism. Some genetically linked disorders involve more than one gland. Although you cannot change your genes, recognizing that you are at risk, taking preventive measures, and seeking early diagnosis and treatment can greatly limit the effects of the condition.

In-Tune

Learning how to be in tune with your body and its processes will greatly assist you towards wellbeing. Understanding the concept of listening to your body or being in-tune, is about observing the signals and messages your body gives you. For example, fatigue, sleep disturbances, appetite changes, weight changes, pain or skin conditions are messages signaling a change in the body. Additionally, observing how your body performs when stressed equips you with a deeper understanding of any changes within your body. For example, when stressed do you develop sleep disturbances, eat more, suffer headaches, weep or become easily confused etc.

Each endocrine gland plays a distinct role in your body; these roles also overlap and therefore affect one another. When one gland is over or under-active, other glands feel the effect. The same goes for you. When part of your endocrine system is sick, you most likely are too. By observing your body and its processes you will become in-tune and identify swiftly the signals and symptoms.

For example, fatigue is one symptom that many endocrine disorders have in common. If you feel unusually tired or can't seem to shake your fatigue, this could be a signal from your body. You can then observe more from your body and look for other signals or look to your environment for changes, which could bring on fatigue i.e. stress, late nights, greater workload etc. Once you've discovered the source of your fatigue whether it's endocrine related or not, there are many remedies you can try under the guidance of a professional both natural and conventional.

Listening to your body, its aches, twinges, feelings of nausea, energy levels etc enables you to hear what may be going on at an inner level and assists you in making correct choices in lifestyle, nutrition, and environmental factors in addition to leading you to a professional if required.

Thoughts and Emotions

"In minds crammed with thoughts, organs clogged with toxins, and bodies stiffened with neglect, there is just no space for anything else."
~ Alison Rose Levy ~

The mind is a veritable storehouse. It is said that 40-50,000 thoughts go through our mind every day. Even if we don't wish to believe this — there are an awful lot of thoughts circulating on a daily basis and this amounts to a pretty powerful broadcast of energy. Most of our thoughts are generated at a sub-conscious level of ingrained patterns of energy such as habitual attitudes, inner dialogue and belief systems. They become affirmations, which determine how we experience the world and help to create our reality. The entire notion of negative emotions and thoughts has far-reaching implications. While it can be difficult to have positive thoughts and attitudes all of the time, everyone can have them most of the time. At the very least, one can monitor them.

Some of you may scoff at the notion of thought and power over the body. I leave you with a thought through the following study. A Yale University professor undertook a study to demonstrate the power of thought. His subject, young male, was suspended on a balanced disk. After instructing the subject to think hard about a difficult mathematical problem it was observed the balanced disk proceeded to tip down where the man's head was positioned. As a result of the blood flow to the brain in the mental exertion it forged enough power to tip the scales. He then instructed the man to think about running, as if going on his daily jog. The balanced disk tipped towards the man's feet as energy followed thought. The professor then asked the subject to repeat the multiplication table and again the disk tipped towards the man's head.

And so the study revealed with thoughts, energy travelled. The blood flow changed direction according to where the thought was directed. Imagine that as a notion in relation to physical conditions or processes such as circulation, digestion and so on. Next time you have cramps of cold feet imagine running and direct the flow of energy to your legs and feet!

Kinesiology is another way of testing power of thoughts and emotions upon the body. Kinesiology is a technical word for muscle testing which is the use of muscle strength as an indicator. The arm (deltoid / shoulder muscle) offers the easiest access for muscle testing. It is not a new fad or undocumented theory; kinesiology has been around for decades and the observations of an American chiropractor, Dr. George Goodheart. It was through his practice that he noticed patient's muscle strength changed noticeably after chiropractic adjustments.

Test This for Yourself:

1. Have your subject stand straight with their right arm relaxed at their side and left arm held straight out, parallel to the floor. (Either arm can be used for testing. If one side becomes fatigued, the other can be used.)

2. Face your subject and place your left hand on their right shoulder to steady them. With your right hand, grasp their extended arm just above the wrist.

3. Instruct the subject to resist as you push down on their arm.

4. Push down on the arm firmly, just hard enough to feel the spring and bounce in the arm. In nearly every case, the muscle will test strong, i.e. the arm will stay resistant to the pressure.

5. Allow your subject to relax their arm for a moment. When ready ask them to think about a time they felt sad and repeat the test using the other arm applying the same firm pressure. In nearly every case, the subject will be unable to resist the pressure and their arm will go down easily. Although you are using the same amount of pressure, the arm goes weak.

6. What has happened? The energy field of the sad event has negatively influenced the energy field of the body and the indicator test muscle (the Deltoid in this case) has lost its strength. The mass has affected the energy field and the altered field has affected the mass.

7. Next have the subject imagine a happy event and repeat the test. Using the same amount of pressure application, you might find that your partner's arm tests strong.

This Following Test Can be Performed with a Larger Group

1. Using the same subject set the audience up with an indicator like thumbs up (positive thought indicator) and thumbs down (negative thought indicator). Turn your subject away from the audience so they cannot see the indicator. Indicate to the audience a 'thumbs up' to direct positive energy towards the subject. Using the same amount of pressure as the previous application, you will discover the subject's arm remains strong.

2. Repeat the test after giving the thumbs down indicator to the audience indicating they direct negative thoughts. In nearly every case, the subject will be unable to resist the pressure and their arm will go down easily. Although you are using the same amount of pressure, the arm goes weak.

This same process can be used to test foods, supplements, items such as watches and even events. With food, supplements and items simply have the subject hold the them in the non-testing hand or close to the thymus and test. If the testing items are non-enhancing for health the arm will weaken, conversely if it is enhancing the arm will remain strong. Testing an event or decision requires you ask the subject to think about the event of decision and test the arm as previously demonstrated.

The Roundabout of Thoughts

Sometimes thoughts simply go round and round. And round and round. It is those persistent thoughts that no matter how hard you try to push-off to another stratosphere they follow you into the night, day and leisure time. Cognitive techniques such as thought stopping and reframing are useful here. This involves being aware and halting the thought before it has the opportunity to take-over or replacing the thought with a positive one. As thoughts and perception are unitary; you can only think one thought at a time, hence substituting a negative thought with a positive one or re-framing with a pleasant memory re-aligns the through structure. If you are thinking about something you enjoy, you cannot simultaneously be thinking of something stressful.

Another way of controlling our emotional states besides changing our attitudes is through our gestures and facial expressions. Two of the most universal of all gestures is a smile and a hug. Smile often, even for no reason, try it and you will see it is difficult to sustain a negative thought. Hug a loved one - do so with a full arm gesture. The most powerful gesture of love is the outstretching of arms to embrace. This is called the 'Madonna' gesture.

To keep a healthy endocrine system and total wellbeing, monitor thoughts and emotions, process that which is necessary for growth and development and 'bin' the rest. If you think you are positive and optimistic ask a close trusted friend for their input — trust what they say and apply the feedback. Often we can be 'immune' to our own negativity or pessimistic outlook and the loving guidance of someone we trust can help shine a torch on our thoughts and emotional behaviors.

Smile, laugh and hug and you will discover negative thoughts simply cannot engage in conjunction with these actions and gestures.

Emotional Counseling

"Emotion always has its roots in the unconscious and manifests itself in the body."
~ **Irene Claremont de Castillejo** ~

Emotions possess the power to lock and store memory in the cellular structures of the human form. This can range from a shock or trauma to grief and sorrow. Emotions such as — hate poisons the cells, grief engulfs our lungs, fear paralyses, anger and rage boils the blood, anxiety churns the stomach, regret and sorrow strip the cells of the spleen and pancreas, jealousy and envy sears through the veins, bitterness and judgement freezes our joints and self-reproach annihilates the spirit.

At the other end of the scale, positive emotions like love, playfulness, joy, contentment and self-mastery have a beneficial effect on good health and they promote healing.

As sentient beings we are designed to feel the entire range of emotions and to express ourselves. Blocking negative emotions isn't the answer to preventing illness. Suppressing emotions will not make them go away. It simply pushes them further into the cauldrons of the body where they lie, festering and releasing toxins into the body's systems.

Considering holistic treatment, the process of releasing past and present conflicts irrespective of the emotions is essential to restoring balance towards wellbeing.

Clearing Emotional Stress with Tapping

Tap the points as illustrated whilst thinking about your health issue or stress. Start at the top of the head and work your way down and onto the hands. Tap with 2 fingers 4 times. At the tender spot, rub firmly, (it will be tender as this area stress emotions) for 10 — 20 seconds.

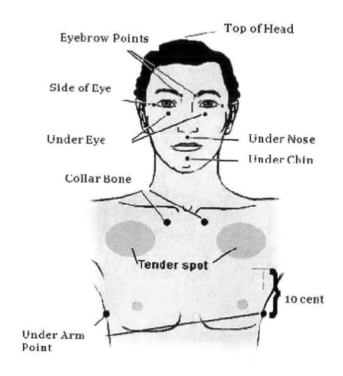

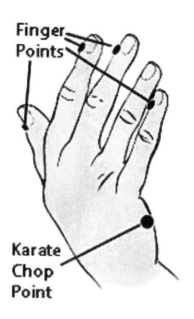

Care of the Soul

"Diseases of the soul are more dangerous and more numerous than those of the body."
~ **Cicero** ~

Care of the soul applies holistic processes towards maintaining equilibrium for the entire body and the endocrine system. Simply, care of the soul is about acknowledging self in harmony with spirit and nature. I am not suggesting one has to adopt a particular religious stance, begin a course in yoga or stand on ones head. What I do suggest however, is that one nurture their being as an entire entity in authenticity and self-honor. What this means is using all the principles of self-care mentioned in this section, committing to it and honoring it. There is virtue in the words 'treat the body as a temple', in doing so we honor our body holistically, we care for our soul.

We can care for our soul in a number of ways:

Meditation
Meditation has been known to decrease stress, alter thought processes and affect the body's life energy in a positive way. Meditation is not just about sitting in the yogi position — meditation is also about other processes that engage all of our senses. When our senses are engaged we become fully immersed – our thoughts are focused, emotions are in check and we are actively participating in our present moment, creating our reality. This can be with any activity, such as gardening, knitting, writing, playing an instrument, cooking or anything that we enjoy and love doing.

Music
Music is another way we can increase our life energy thus

maintaining a healthy endocrine system. There has long been an association between longevity and musical conductors. It is well documented that major music conductors have lived and are enjoying exceptionally long, healthy lives. Our bodies have a pulse and so does music. In a healthy state, we are in touch with our 'inner pulse'. Surrounded by the right sounds, we can be invigorated, energized and balanced.

Throughout the ages the therapeutic value of music has been recognized and respected. It has been demonstrated clinically that music adds to our general health and wellbeing. However, not all music benefits our wellbeing. Rock music with the characteristics of the anapestic beat switches off the thymus and endocrine systems and has a detrimental effect on our wellbeing, immune system and equilibrium.

Extensive research postulates the anapestic beat [two short beats, a long beat, then a pause] used by many rock musicians is the exact opposite of our heart and arterial rhythms thereby causing an immediate loss of body strength. Furthermore, rock music contains harmonic dissonance and melodic discord, which sends a vibrational energy to our inner organs creating dissonance and discord.

Nature's music such as the sound of the ocean, waterfalls, rain, wind or birds bear a similar rhythm to our body. No guessing why leisure pursuits in nature is so beneficial to our wellbeing and relaxation.

Doing What You Love To Do

Participating in any activity that nurtures your entire being will care for the soul and assist in maintaining a healthy endocrine system. This can be anything that you choose to do and reflects your inner nurturing processes, maybe reading a book, sitting in the sun, singing, spending time with loved ones, simply doing just what one wants to do.

Visualize Yourself into Good Health

"The pictures in our minds have power. They are not just passing through."
~ **Marilyn King, U.S. Olympic pentathlete** ~

Dr Phineas P Quimby mental and spiritual healer said the imagination is the most powerful faculty of the human mind ... what the mind images becomes experience and fact.

That means, though the conscious use of our imagination we can produce wonderful changes in the body and in every area of our life. Thus, the imagination becomes a powerful tool for healing.

We are always creating through the imagination. We are always creating through visualization and affirmation. What we speak we affirm, people who always talk about sickness, or poverty are usually surrounded by it.

The power of vision is about using the power of the imagination to create an image. It is a state of awareness in which we are not thinking about, analyzing or figuring out our experiences, but actually experiencing them directly. Results come much quicker when we picture what we want, rather than just vaguely thinking about it.

One of the first steps towards improved health is to definitely picture it. Generalities do not heal; they lack substance. Vague hopes and indefinite goals are not convincing to the mind. A clear cut picture of your goal motivates both mind and body in the healing process. Picture yourself healthy — doing things you haven't been able to do. Imagine in your mind how you want to look. Judge Thomas Troward said once, "Once you have seen the result you wish to attain, you have already willed a means that will take you to that result."

There are 20 times as many nerves running from the eye to the brain than from the ears to the brain. The higher glands — pituitary, pineal and hypothalamus — are instrumental in the visualization processes. Between the eyes is a ganglionic nerve center which when deliberately quickened will set into operation your imaging mind power. This is a point of expression for a set of tissues that extend back into the brain and connect with an imaging or picture making function near the root of the optic nerve.

Always visualize as if it's actually happened right now. Make it real in your mind, make it detailed. Enter the role and become it. Make the commitment to use this vision daily, as if it were already created now. Know that every time you visualize your dream you change or reverse in-built programming which may interfere with your successful achievement.

(Scientific research reveals that it takes 21 days to re-program our brain patterns.)

A university in the United States conducted the following study on the effects of Creative Visualization. A basketball team was selected and split into 3 groups and were to be tested after a period of 1 month on their ability to score baskets:

1. First group were asked to do no practice at all.

2. Second group were asked to mentally practice for half an hour per day — shooting and scoring.

3. Third group practiced for half-hour every day.

4. After one month all 3 groups were tested. Group 1 - group showed no improvement. Group 2 - showed 20% improvement and Group 3 showed 20% improvement

Affirm Yourself into Good Health

"Affirm what you know to be true in your heart, and you will create that reality."
~ Anon ~

To affirm means to make firm. There is little mystery about how and why affirmations work once the principle is understood. An affirmation is simply a spoken declaration in the present tense, which creates a desired reality. Every day we affirm — we self talk — we speak and it manifests. When we affirm statements regarding our health and body, we reinforce a message. Sayings such as — "I'm sick and tired," "it makes my blood boil," "he/she is a pain in the neck," "I am going crazy." And there are the family curses — "we Jones's die young," "cancer runs in the family," "I can't help it, I am genetically pre-disposed," "the females/males in this family all suffer from this." When we speak of disease, we invariably attract it. Statements such as these affirm and attract a state of being in ill health.

Indeed every word is recorded in the body. Our words become our flesh. Every word when spoken vibrates throughout our entire body and reverberates within each cell. Repetition of words fixes itself to the cellular structure and becomes a force.

Every Day, in Every Way, I'm Getting Better and Better
Power is released by stating words which exude life, health, vitality and wellbeing. The body can be renewed, even trans-formed through the spoken world, through affirming. Words do indeed have power; every time we affirm something we send a message to the universe, to our cells, to our brain. Émile Coué de Châtaigneraie (February 26, 1857 — July 2, 1926) French psychol-ogist and pharmacist introduced a method of self-improvement based on optimistic autosuggestion. A more familiar term used

today is affirmation or mantra.

Émile coined the phrase — or mantra-like - autosuggestion, "Every day, in every way, I'm getting better and better" — and is known as the Couéism or the Coué method. This method is similar to regular practices of affirmation used today by many therapists. It centers upon a routine repetition of a particular expression according to a specified ritual, in the absence of any sort of allied mental imagery, at regular times of the day. This process effects a change in consciousness but initially demands a change in our unconscious thought, which can only be achieved by using our imagination.

Even during treatment either through medication or under supervision from a medical practitioner, we can utilize effectively this processes of affirmation. Coué believed in the effects of medication. But he also believed that our mental state is able to affect and even amplify the action of these medications. He believed in certain cases he could improve the efficiency of a given medicine by praising its effectiveness to the patient. He realized that those patients to whom he praised the medicine had a noticeable improvement when compared to patients to whom he said nothing. By consciously using autosuggestion, he observed that his patients could cure themselves more efficiently by replacing their "thought of illness" with a new "thought of cure."

By repeating words or images enough times causes the subconscious to absorb them which in effect changes the conscious mind. Simply repeat the affirmation or mantra — "Every day, in every way, I'm getting better and better," and allow for improvement. Catch yourself using negative affirmations and replace it with —"Every day, in every way, I'm getting better and better."

Herbs and Foods for a Healthy Endocrine

"The wise man should consider that health is the greatest of human blessings. Let food be your medicine."
~ **Hippocrates** ~

Supporting the endocrine system via nutritional methods has an almost immediate effect. There is much we can do at this level through awareness and knowledge of food properties and how they interact with the endocrine glands.

Hypothalamus

- Olive leaf extract, brahma, brassica family (cabbage, collards, kale, broccoli, cauliflower, brussels' sprouts, mustard, turnips, radishes, etc.)

Pineal

- Consuming foods high in melatonin or the melatonin precursor tryptophan, such as oats, sweet corn, rice, ginger, tomatoes, bananas, barley, Japanese radish, spirulina, soy, cottage cheese, chicken meat/liver, turkey, pepitas, almonds and peanuts.

- Cherries, a little miracle fruit is also a natural source of melatonin, so if you are finding that your sleep is disturbed then add some cherries to your diet to help put you into a peaceful slumber.

Pituitary

- High amounts of bromines found in melons and celery

enhance the growth hormones.

Thyroid

- Kelp helps to replenish iodine supplies. Kelp also helps to stimulate cancer fighting T-cells, thereby strengthening the immune system.

- Kelp also helps to protect against heavy metals and ionising radiation by binding in the intestinal tract and preventing their absorption.

Thymus

- Vitamin E protects the thymus gland and white blood cells from damage — particularly important in protecting the immune system from damage during times of oxidative stress.

- Zinc is considered one of the most important nutrients for the immune system. It is necessary for healthy antibody, white blood cell, thymus gland and hormone function.

- Immune building herbs such as, echinacea also known as the 'prairie doctor' because it promotes the production of white blood cells which then destroy invading bacteria, microbes and virus infections.

- Medicinal mushrooms such as shitake, reishi, maitake, cordyceps, coriolus versicolor and agaricus blazei have the ability to stimulate all white blood cells as well as provide many other positive immune system effects. These ancient medicinal mushrooms are extremely powerful immune system boosters that are my prime choice for the immune system.

- Other foods which support are immune-system-stimu-lating are - onions, garlic, ginger, bitter melon, whole grains, legumes, fish, salmon, tuna, mackerel, sardines, nuts and seeds, sprouts, dark green leafy vegetable, turmeric and fruits. Eat plenty of orange, yellow and green vegetables to enhance immune system responses.

- Balanced levels of protein to maintain good immune system function and tissue repair.

- Aim for organic produce or use a product like the Lotus Sanitiser or hydrogen peroxide (at a low percentage) to remove harmful pesticides.

Pancreas

- Liquorice tea helps to balance hypoglycaemia.

- Foods loaded with vitamin C, carotenoids, folate and fiber. Such as dark, leafy greens like spinach, kale Brassica family such as broccoli and brussel sprouts, orange-yellow vegetables such as squash, sweet potatoes, and carrots.

- Foods that naturally contain magnesium, potassium or sodium will help to stimulate the correct functioning of this gland.

Adrenals

- Parsley root and licorice root is an energizer.

- Vitamin B complex and vitamin C which help to restore

adrenals after stressful periods along with bioflavonoid and zinc.

- Useful herbs for adrenal exhaustion are — oat straw, valerian, vervain, royal jelly, skullcap, lavender, peppermint, passion flower, lady's slipper, hops and chamomile.

- Useful vitamins and nutrients are iodine, magnesium, manganese, phosphorous, and sulphur.

- Foods which exhaust the adrenals must be avoided, such as excessive amounts of coffee or caffeine drinks, tea, sugar, alcohol, and drugs.

Gonads

- Progesterone and testosterone are both found in sarsaparilla root and in ginseng.

- Natural hormones around available in herbs and plants:
  ~ Genitstein from soybeans
  ~ Prunetin from prunes
  ~ Diadzein from soybeans
  ~ Formononetin for red clover
  ~ Coumarin from alfalfa
  ~ Estriol from Willow catkins

- Progesterone and estrogen hormones are found in: carrots, soybeans, licorice root, blessed thistle herb, wheat, barley, potatoes, apple, cherry plums, garlic, wheat germ, rice bran.

Schuessler Cell Salts

"Restoration of the cell, and thereby of the body, will result from restoration of the deficit of the inorganic salts."
~ **Dr Schuessler** ~

19th century German physician, Dr Schuessler, discovered 12 mineral salts vital to restoring and maintaining health. These salts — *cell salts* — are constitutes of every cell in the body, an imbalance of which results in ill-health and give rise to specific symptoms. They work on bring about homeostasis at a cellular level thus work towards sustainable health.

The Twelve Cell Salts

Calc Fluor - 'Elasticity Salt'
Present in bones, tooth enamel, muscle tissue, blood vessels.
Imbalance results in: muscular weakness, impaired circulation, eczema, wrinkles, osteoporosis, cracked skin, poor teeth, hemorrhoids, varicose veins, inability to cope.
Evident as swelling or cracks on the tongue.
Symptoms are worse in damp weather.

Calc Phos - 'Nutrient Tonic'
Present in bones, teeth, connective tissue, blood corpuscles.
Imbalance results in: impaired digestion, chilblains, colic, anemia, osteoporosis, growing pains.
Evident as numbness or pimples on the tongue.
Symptoms are worse in humidity, motion, water.

Calc Sulph - 'Cell Healer, Blood Purifier'
Present in the liver.
Imbalance results in: vertigo, acne, kidney disorders, boils,

frontal headaches, slow healing wounds.
Evident as yellow clay-like coating at base of the tongue.
Symptoms are worse by water.

Ferr Phos- 'First Aid Salt - Oxygen Carrier'
Present in hemoglobin.
Imbalance results in, hot dry skin, thirst, redness.
Evident as swollen, red, inflamed tongue.
Symptoms are worse for cold air, motion or exertion.

Kali Mur- 'Blood Conditioner'
Present in every tissue in the body except bone.
Imbalance results in: catarrh, congestion, bronchitis, glandular
    swellings, sinus, jaundice, eustachian tubes, eczema, allergies.
Evident as white or gray coating of the tongue.
Symptoms are worse for motion, eating pastry, rich fatty foods.

Kali Phos - 'Nerve Nutrient'
Present in nerve tissue and all body fluids.
Imbalance results in: skin problems, paralysis, shingles, fear,
    tired, nervous exhaustion, depression, irritability.
Evident as dark mustard color coating on the tongue.
Symptoms are worse for cold, noise, mental exertion, worry.

Kali Sulph - 'Skin Salt'
Present in the cells of the skin and mucous lining of all organs.
Imbalance results in: catarrh, skin eruptions, dry scaling skin,
    dandruff, loss of hair, psoriasis, athlete's foot, anxiety, brittle
    nails.
Evident as yellow coating on the tongue.
Symptoms are worse for stuffy rooms.

Mag Phos - 'Nerve Stabilizer'
Present in muscles, nerves, bone, brain, and spine.

Imbalance results in: spasmodic pains, cramps, neuralgia, flatulence, hunger pains, hiccups, twitching.

Evident as yellowish green or a dirty brown coating on the tongue.

Symptoms worse for cold air and water, lying on the right side.

Nat Mur - 'Fluid Balancer & Water Distributor'

Present in every cell and fluid in the body.

Imbalance results in: dryness or excessive moisture, eczema, shingles, loss of taste or smell.

Evident as slimy small bubbles of frothy saliva on the tongue.

Symptoms worse for heat, closed rooms, thunder.

Nat Phos - 'Acid Neutralizer'

Present in the blood muscle, nerve, brain cells and the fluid between cells.

Imbalance results in: kidney or bladder disorders, jaundice, arthritis, diabetes, gout, sour breath, cholesterol, cravings, body odor, worms, acidity.

Evident as thick, golden yellow coating on the tongue.

Symptoms worse for mental and physical exertion and changes in weather.

Nat Sulph - 'Water Eliminator'

The liver salt.

Imbalance results in: bilious headaches, diarrhea, sluggish liver, gallstones, fluid retention, jaundice, digestive disorders, bitter taste, vomiting of bile.

Evident as dirty, yellow coating on the tongue.

Symptoms are worse for damp, wet weather and from lying on left side.

Silica - 'Toxic Eliminator'

Present in the blood, skin, hair, nails, bones.

Imbalance results in: body odor, cataracts, sty's, inability to connect thoughts, boils, hair loss, pimples, dry skin & hair, noise or light sensitivity.

Evident as ulcers on the tongue.

Symptoms are worse for night air, cold, touch, drafts.

Bach Flower Remedies

"I want to make it as simple as this: I am hungry, I will go and pull a lettuce form the garden; I am frightened and ill, I will take a dose of Mimulus."

~ Dr. Edward Bach ~

There are 38 Bach Flower Remedies developed by Dr Edward Bach (1886-1936). He believed that negative emotions cause illness, and that flowers prepared in a specific manner can fight these negative emotions. "Instead of looking at symptoms, we look at the emotional outlook of people," explains Bach, "the remedies are basically positive energy pushing out the negative."

Each remedy correlates to a set of emotional symptoms which affect the endocrine system at an energetic level. By restoring harmony to the body via the emotions a vibratory frequency sets off a chain reaction at a cellular level and assists in restoring homeostasis.

There are seven general categories of emotions that Bach flower remedies target, including:

1. Uncertainty
2. Lack of interest in daily life
3. Loneliness
4. Hypersensitivity
5. Despair
6. Caring too much about others
7. Fear

Bach's theory revealed that each individual had a specific personality type and corresponding flower. These he described as the twelve personality types. The asterisk * indicates one of the twelve personality types, commonly known as the twelve healers.

Agrimony - mental torture behind a cheerful face

Aspen - fear of unknown things

Beech — intolerance, criticism

Centaury - the inability to say 'no'

Cerato - lack of trust in one's own decisions

Cherry Plum - fear of the mind giving way

Chestnut Bud - failure to learn from mistakes

Chicory - selfish, possessive love

Clematis - dreaming of the future without working in the present

Crab Apple - the cleansing remedy, also for self-hatred

Elm - overwhelmed by responsibility

Gentian - discouragement after a setback

Gorse - hopelessness and despair

Heather - self-centerdness and self-concern

Holly - hatred, envy and jealousy

Honeysuckle - living in the past, wishing things could be the way they used to be

Hornbeam - tiredness at the thought of doing something

Impatiens - impatience

Larch - lack of confidence

Mimulus - fear of known things

Mustard - deep gloom for no reason

Oak - the plodder who keeps going past the point of exhaustion

Olive - exhaustion following mental or physical effort

Pine - guilt

Red Chestnut - over-concern for the welfare of loved ones

Rock Rose - terror and fright

Rock Water - self-denial, rigidity and self-repression

Scleranthus - inability to choose between alternatives

Star of Bethlehem - shock

Sweet Chestnut - extreme mental anguish, when everything has been tried and there is no light left

Vervain - over-enthusiasm
Vine - dominance and inflexibility
Walnut - protection from change and unwanted influences
Water Violet - pride and aloofness
White Chestnut - unwanted thoughts and mental arguments
Wild Oat - uncertainty over one's direction in life
Wild Rose - drifting, resignation, apathy
Willow - self-pity and resentment

The Twelve Healers — Personality Types

Agrimony
The Agimony personality tends to hide more deeply rooted pain or ailments behind a cheerful façade, both inwardly and outwardly. They may make light of their own suffering, or try to ignore it all together, when really there are patterns and feelings which need to be addressed for personal growth and healing. These individuals may have been raised in strict environments, which may not have allowed the expression of such troubles. Agrimony flower essence can help them find inner peace, by allowing the connection to true inner conditions, acceptance of these conditions, and subsequent transformation.

Centaury
This personality finds it difficult to say no. The result is devalued self, and the spreading thin of personal energies. There is the recurrent theme of personal boundaries being overstepped, because the will to create and enforce those boundaries is weak. Centaury flower essence strengthens the value of one's self, supporting the notion that one's life in and of itself is of impor-tance. The idea that one must truly be honoring and respectful to one's self first, before others can be served, is reinforced — It is then that personal healing can finally be initiated as a powerful force.

Cerato

Cerato personality types do not trust their own hearts, minds or instincts; instead they seek the advice of others, and rely on this advice to direct their lives. This almost certainly creates an imbalance, for it is only by honestly listening to our own inner voice that we may walk the path to true physical and emotional wellness. While seeking advice is certainly important in most of life's circumstances, the Cerato type uses this advice as a crutch. Cerato flower essence will encourage one to listen to one's own inner wisdom and facilitate spiritual growth in this respect.

Chicory

The Chicory personality tends towards self-pity, and the 'nobody appreciates me' attitude. A guise of seemingly loving behavior can be used to manipulate others into feeding somewhat selfish needs. The Chicory essence is considered important for clearing loving energy pathways so they may be directed outward and given freely. May be particularly helpful with children who have a pattern of negative behavior for demanding attention.

Clematis

The Clematis personality type is a dreamy one; there is insufficient interest in the immediate moment of daily life. The individual may have a strong inner life — the abilities to dream, visualize and imagine are well developed, but the manifestation into the physical world is not strong. Clematis can help bring a warmth to the bodily incarnation, such that the individual can channel their great gifts into the here and now.

Gentian

The Gentian personality type is easily discouraged when setbacks occur. They may live with an omnipresent feeling that things are not going well, and may doubt the possibility of their own healing. Gentian can bring about a more positive outlook —

perhaps with the feeling that one is 'good enough'. When things do not go exactly as planned, instead of being overwhelmed and disheartened, one can see the lessons in the circumstance, perhaps rebounding with more wisdom and strength than before.

Impatiens

As the name of the flower implies, this personality has a tendency toward impatience; these individuals have difficulty with the flow of time. Their minds are often far ahead of the present moment, and with this they will deny themselves full immersion in the beauty around them. The individual needing Impatiens may be truly lonely, always being ahead of those subtle human exchanges which bring the richness to our collective human experience. Many find Impatiens to be a relatively 'fast acting' flower essence, feeling more at ease within minutes of essence use.

Mimulus

This personality is assailed by known fears in everyday life. They can be hypersensitive to common events which will elicit an out-of-proportion fear response. The fear may be found in the physical body centerd in the solar plexus, which may churn with anxiety. Mimulus flower essence helps bring courage to these individuals, bringing the strength of the higher self to the personality so that they may find joy and exuberance in their lives.

Rock Rose

This is the flower essence for great fear. Unlike Mimulus, which is indicated more for a fear which manifests as being timid, Rock Rose personality is in a state of terror. It is often indicated in traumatic events (as a component of Rescue Remedy) or for specific instances where a reaction of overwhelming fear is inhibiting further growth or healing. If one has been diagnosed with a life threatening illness, for example, and one is overcome with the fear of death, this fear will inhibit any healing process that may take place. Rock Rose brings courage to those most in need.

Scleranthus
The personality in need of Scleranthus flower essence is marked by indecision, confusion and hesitation, often wavering between two choices. This inability to decide the best course of actions for one's self can be physically and emotionally draining - this mental energy is used repeatedly examining a situation rather than manifesting the best choice. The world can be a difficult place for such individuals, as there are limitless possibilities in which to get lost, never really making headway. Scleranthus will help these individuals define themselves and their world, summoning the strength to form an inner resolve. This allows a great release of energy to be happy and manifest one's chosen work.

Vervain
The lesson of the Vervain personality is one of balance. The individual in need of Vervain may be extreme, over-bearing, and very strong — perhaps inflexible — in their ways. Though their energies are high, the single-minded efforts of the Vervain type can result in stress, when given situations where flexibility is required. This is where the mind-body connection can be lost; the mind can be so strongly committed to a particular action, it may no longer consider the long-term effects to the physical being. Vervain flower essence brings grounding and earthly balance, allowing these strong-willed individuals the flexibility necessary to manifest their great intentions and efforts.

Water Violet
The Water Violet personality learns about opening of the heart.

Those in need of this essence may be functioning quite effectively in society and within their familial relationships; however, the deepest parts of these bonds are avoided. Whether due to childhood experiences, karma brought to this life from the past, or other situations, the individual has constructed a barrier preventing full integration with the human family. The true warmth of love and companionship should be utilized to further one's growth — Water Violet flower essence supports this transformation.

Color Therapies

"The art of healing comes from nature, not from the physician. Therefore the physician must start from nature, with an open mind."
~ Philipus Aureolus Paracelsus ~

Color therapy is the use of color to produce beneficial or healing effects at an energetic level. Color can be applied through foods, crystals, color swatches, lights, clothing and visualizations. Working at an energetic level color restores harmony to imbalance as well as restores depleted color energies from the body's systems. Each of the chakras, aura and glands respond to a color frequency.

Color Spectrum

Red
Gonads, bones, muscles of the lower back, sciatic nerve, hips, buttocks, lower bowels, legs, ankles, feet, prostrate gland, blood, and appendix.

> *Layer of the Aura* — Etheric
> *Chakra* — Muladhara
> *Endocrine* — Gonads

Red is a powerful healing agent for healing diseases of the blood and circulation. It will warm cold areas to reduce pain and drying up weeping sores or wounds. Use it when you are low in energy or when you feel apathetic on a mental, emotional spiritual or physical level. Beneficial at times when you know you are in for a hectic day, and you want that extra boost.

Not recommended for fever, wounds, bruises, hyperactivity, high blood pressure or aggressive types. Can also bring out eruptions if lying dormant. Red should not be worn for long periods of time.

Orange
Adrenals, body fluids, kidneys and bladder, lymphatic system, reproductive system, fat deposits, skin, pelvis.

Layer of the Aura — Emotional
Chakra— Svadhisthana
Endocrine —Adrenals

It is used to increase immunity, enhance sexual potency, to help in all digestive ailments, chest, and kidney diseases. Its many therapeutic qualities include gallstones, chest conditions, arthritis and repressed creativity. Use orange when you cannot enjoy your own thought process or you lack joy in your life. It uplifts and gives back the energy you lose through putting into being unhappy.

Orange is a great emotional stimulant. It connects us to our senses and helps to remove inhibitions and makes us independent and social.

Yellow
Pancreas, spleen, nerves and muscular energies, liver and intestines, cellular repair, umbilical area.

Layer of the Aura — Mental
Chakra— Manipura
Endocrine —Pancreas

As it is the color of intellect, it is used for mental stimulation helps to bring clarification and perspective. It is good for clearing a foggy head and increases awareness.

Yellow has a cleansing affect on the skin and those who suffer skin disorders will find that bright, clear shades of yellow in personal clothing are very beneficial. Yellow relates to the spleen and life force energy. Not to be used for insomnia, over-excitement, or in nausea or diarrhoea.

Green and Turquoise

Thymus gland, immune system, central nervous system, heart and lungs, automatic processes such as sweating.

> *Layer of the Aura* — Astral
> *Chakra* — Anahata
> *Endocrine* — Thymus

Green is the color of harmony and balance and is good for tired nerves as it brings balance to the emotions and a feeling of calmness. Green is a good general healing color because it stimulates growth so it is good for broken bones, re-growth of tissue of all kinds.

Blue

Thyroid and parathyroid, throat and neck, blood and circulation, spine and nervous system, and temperature control.

> *Layer of the Aura* — Causal
> *Chakra* — Vishuddha
> *Endocrine* — Thyroid and parathyroid

Blue has a pacifying effect on the nervous system and brings great relaxation, serenity and harmony. Ideal for sleep problems, and hyper-active children and also assists with feverish conditions, it will help stop bleeding and it will help with nervous irritations.

Too much blue could leave you cold, depressed and sorrowful. Not to be used in cold conditions and low metabolic types, paralysis, low blood pressure or depression.

Violet or Purple
Pituitary, all the senses, muscular responses and control and coordination, head.

Layer of the Aura — Celestial
Chakra — Ajna
Endocrine — Pituitary

The colors of equilibrium, it helps with overall spiritual healing. Excellent for mental and nervous problems and will assist with rheumatism and inflammations. Purple and violet are anti-bacterial and can help replenish and rebuild as it acts like a tonic for the body.

A keyword for violet is dignity and works on feelings of self-worth and can be used when feeling low in esteem. Violet is useful to strengthen the body's ability to assimilate minerals.

Not to be used for depression, negative conditions, low vitality.

Magenta
Pineal and hypothalamus, entire nervous system.

Layer of the Aura — Ketheric
Chakra — Sahasrara
Endocrine — Pineal and Hypothalamus

Purifies our thoughts and feelings giving us inspiration in all undertakings. This energy connects us to our spiritual self bringing guidance, wisdom and inner strength. Enhances artistic talent and creativity.

Magenta is letting go. That is letting go of old patterns in your emotional, mental, spiritual and physical life. Use it where change is needed. Particularly the change required when embarking on a new spiritual path. Those who wish to serve humanity will find Magenta uplifting. Magenta induces spirituality, it brings with it a recognition of spiritual energies, and unconditional love.

If you have a tendency towards over-exertion, try wearing magenta colors. Particularly helpful when thoughts go round and round in your head. Not to be used in feverish, excited or plethoric states.

Color Methods

Using the above descriptions we can apply color healing to our everyday lifestyles through the food we eat, clothes we wear and other techniques such as color breathing and visualization.

Color Breathing

Color breathing can be done anywhere. First, lie or sit in a comfortable position. Become totally relaxed, block out distractions and noises. Think of a time when you felt totally happy, content and peaceful. Visualize the color needed or hold a colored piece of cotton, material, silk scarf or piece of clothing near you.

If you are having trouble seeing the color, place the colored item over your eyes. Breathe the color in through your nostrils or the solar plexus (lower chest area). Direct it to the area of the body that needs the healing. Imagine the color flowing down to this area and feel its healing essence. Say to yourself that this area is getting better and better every moment and improving all the time. Know this and believe this!

Do this exercise for 10 to 15 minutes at any time of the day. It is a great therapy to do in the morning before starting the day, or in the evening before retiring for bed. Imagine the appropriate color permeating your entire being and always reaffirm greater health and well-being.

Colored Clothing

Wearing the right color clothing can be beneficial for uplifting the spirit or minor disturbances. Even dying your hair different colors has an effect on your physical and mental health.

Colored Foods

Eating different colored foods also enhances healing. Red, orange and yellow foods have an alkaline and stimulating effect, similar to the colors. Green foods tend to be neutral and balancing. Blue, indigo and violet foods have a calming effect.

Color Healing Devices

There are a number of different color healing devices that you can purchase including color therapy glasses, full spectrum light devices and other chromo therapy devices.

Acupressure Points and the Endocrine

"Don't let your mind bully your body into believing it must carry the burden of its worries."
~ **Astrid Alauda** ~

Seeking out a professional for alternative therapies such as reflexology, massage and acupressure can greatly assist in maintaining a healthy endocrine system and enhance the function of our *Personal Tuning Fork*.

However, we can perform some functions on a regular basis ourselves. The following diagrams demonstrate various points on our face, feet and ear which if gently massaged can assist our body's process, the endocrine system and the function of your *Personal Tuning Fork*.

The Adrenal/Stress Release Button

The Face

The Ear

Ear tapping points – balances the entire endocrine system

For all over well being, massage both ears in turn by taking the entire ear between the fingers an thumb. Start at the top and work down as hard as you can tolerate 4 times. You should feel a tingling and the effect will be evident in the facial muscles in the face.

The Feet

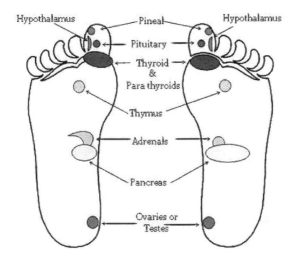

The Hands

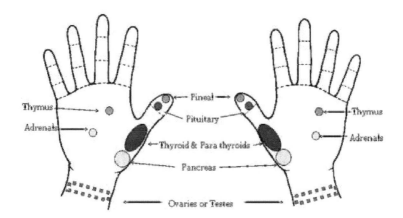

Yoga for the Endocrine

"Every human being is the author of his own health or disease."
~ Buddha ~

Hypothalamus

Sahasrara - Crown Chakra

1. Position a folded blanket under the shoulders. The head and neck should be off the blanket.
2. Lie on the back.
3. Using the abdominal muscles, lift the legs over the head until the toes touch the floor behind the head.
4. Interlace the fingers behind your back and straighten the arms.
5. Roll the shoulders under one at a time.
6. The hips should be aligned over the shoulders.
7. To come out, roll out of the pose slowly, one vertebra at a time, keeping the legs straight and feet together.

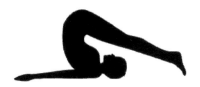

Pineal

Sahasrara - Crown Chakra

1. Position yourself on your hands and knees with the wrists underneath the shoulders and the knees underneath the hips.
2. Curl the toes under and push back raising the hips and straightening the legs.
3. Spread the fingers and ground down from the forearms into the fingertips.
4. Outwardly rotate the upper arms broadening the collar-

bones.

5. Let the head hang, move the shoulder blades away from the ears towards the hips.

6. Engage the quadriceps strongly to take the weight off the arms, making this a resting pose.

7. Rotate the thighs inward, keep the tail high and sink your heels towards the floor.

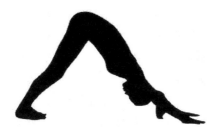

Pituitary

Ajna - Third Eye Chakra

1. Lie down on your back, inhale as you bend your knees and bring them towards your chest

2. Exhale and swing your legs upwards so that your hips lift off the floor

3. Using your hands, support your lower back as you raise your legs into the air

4. Keep your legs as straight as possible

5. Breath in and out for as long as comfortable

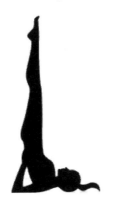

Thyroid Parathyroid's

Vishuddha - Throat Chakra

1. Lie on your back.
2. Come up onto your elbows.
3. Slide your body towards the back of the mat while keeping your forearms in place and puffing up your chest.
4. Drop the crown of your head back to the floor, opening your throat.
5. To come out, press strongly into your forearms and raise your head off the floor.
6. Release your upper body to the floor.

Thymus

Anahata - Heart Chakra

1. Come up onto your knees. Take padding under your knees if they are sensitive.
2. Draw your hands up the side of your body as you start to open your chest.
3. Reach your hands back one at a time to grasp your heels.
4. Bring your hips forward so that they are over your knees.
5. Let your head come back, opening your throat.

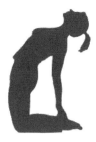

Pancreas

Manipura - Solar Plexus Chakra

1. Place yourself on all fours and pull your stomach towards the floor to arch your back
2. Inhale and raise your head
3. Exhale as you push your stomach away from the floor, rounding your back, pushing your head down
4. Repeat 5 times if possible

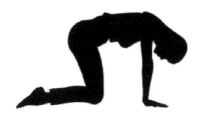

Spleen/Kidneys

Manipura - Solar Plexus Chakra

1. Lie on the stomach, taking a blanket under the hips as padding.
2. Reach the hands back and take hold of the ankles.
3. On an inhale, draw the torso and legs up off the floor simultaneously.
4. If you can, bring the thighs to rest on the floor

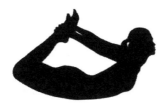

Adrenals

Svadhisthana - Sacral Chakra

1. Lay face down and have your hands next to your chest, elbows bent in beside the body, palms flat.
2. Inhale and focus on lengthening from the tail bone as you raise the chest off the floor. Press your hands, legs and lower pelvis gently into floor.
3. Keep your chin down slightly as you lengthen through the back and front of the neck. Keep your shoulders down as you draw your shoulder blades into your back
4. Relax your back.
5. Exhale and slowly lower.
6. Rest and repeat x 5

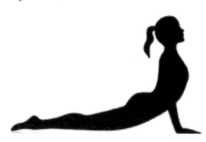

Gonads

Muladhara - Base Chakra

1. Lying flat on your back, hands palm down by your sides, bend your knees and bring your feet close to your bottom making sure your feet are parallel on the yoga mat.
2. Pressing your feet firmly against the ground, lift your hips up towards the ceiling.
3. Interlace your fingers under you, straighten your arms, and press them down on to the mat to raise your back and chest higher.
4. Roll your shoulders and draw your chest towards your chin.
5. Stay and breath

6. Release the pose, by releasing your hands back into the palm down position beside you, then bringing the your upper, middle then lower back and hips down. Knees are still bent

7. Allow your knees to touch and rest.

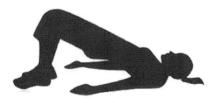

Total

1. Drop the knees to the floor.
2. Spread the knees as wide as the mat, keeping the big toes touching.
3. Bring the belly to rest between the thighs and the forehead to the floor.
4. There are two possible arm variations: Either stretch the arms in front of you with the palms toward the floor or bring the arms back alongside the thighs with the palms facing upwards. Do whichever feel more comfortable to you.

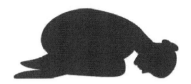

Total

1. Standing upright bring your arms out to the side and up.
2. Press the palms together, keep the arms straight and take the gaze up toward your thumbs.
3. Slide the shoulder blades down the back.
4. Maintain your alignment.

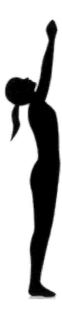

Bring your palms together and use your middle and index fingers to lightly touch the third eye point located between your eyebrows. Breathe deeply as you hold this point for balancing your endocrine system.

In assessing the chakras and their functions and combining the symptomatic picture with the symptomatic picture of the individual glands and meridians, one can develop a holistic and greater picture towards self-care and the practice of holistic applications in balancing both endocrine gland and chakra.

Personal Tuning Fork Daily Tuning Guide

Implementing any of these suggestions greatly enhances your well-being and ability to maintain sustainable health towards homeostasis.

A creative approach to selecting a the most appropriate one for your daily needs is to think of a number from 1 - 27. Random selection can open up the intuition to speak.

1. Tap the thymus three or four times a day to activate it and reduce the effects of stress. This will kick start your entire endocrine system
2. Take frequent energy breaks in your day and ensure you look at a pleasant scene.
3. Listen to revitalizing music
4. Allow your body to absorb the sounds of nature, birds or running water
5. Place your tongue on the 'Centering Button'
6. Apply gentle pressure to the 'Stress Release Button' located 3 finger widths below navel
7. Smile as often as you can. Do it several times a day as an exercise
8. Think positively, affirm those thoughts, praise yourself and walk proud ·
9. Dwell on positive thoughts - love, faith, trust, gratitude, and courage
10. Eat well, drink plenty of water and supplement with herbs and minerals if you skip meals
11. Get to know your body, develop an intuitive knowing regarding its rhythms and needs
12. Breathe deep into and expanding the belly
13. Laugh long and frequently
14. Nurture your soul by honoring its needs and requests

15. Do nothing - rest, restore, revitalize
16. Massage your feet and the acupressure points at the end of the day
17. Rub the ears for all over wellbeing or for a quick burst of energy
18. Apply gentle pressure to the endocrine points on your face and head first thing in the morning or at the end of the day. (Refer to chapter on Acupressure Points and the Endocrine)
19. Pranayama nostril breathing technique
20. Monitor the Triple Warmer Meridian
21. Balance the chakras. (Refer to the chapter on the Chakras)
22. Balance the meridians. (Refer to the chapter on the Meridians)
23. Give yourself a definite wake up and sleep time. This helps you feel well, sleep soundly, and awake refreshed
24. Monitor the consumption of sugar, caffeine, and other stimulants you use. People who are stressed almost always begin to use stimulants as a boost. Stimulants put the body under even more stress. Eating more raw foods and vegetables can help your body deal with stress instead of increasing it
25. Exercise three times a week. Enjoyable exercise, in moderation, reduces stress. It will make you feel better right away
26. Dancing, listening to music, reading, working on a craft, playing a musical instrument, meditation, and biofeedback also relieve stress
27. Balance both sides of the hemisphere. Techniques such as reading poetry aloud, marching on the spot exaggerating the arm movements to a full cross swing, alternating humming a few bars of a song - any song - with counting 1, 2, 3.
28. Hug someone today

29. Create something today. Can be as simple as a new recipe, a paper airplane or a garden bed

30. Break your routine. Do something different or change the way you currently do something. This could be taking a different route to work or changing a daily habit

31. Cleanse the aura (refer to chapter on the aura)

32. Maintain acid/alkaline balance within the body to ensure your body's pH levels are balanced

33. Practice Brahmari (Humming Bee) Breathing. Place the index finger and middle finger on the area between the eyes and just above the bridge of the nose. Sit comfortably, relax and close the eyes. Begin to hum like a bee on the long outward breath. As you hum you will notice a vibration in the bones of our head. If the hum is low you will feel it more in the jaw whereas a higher hum brings the vibration up into the cheek bones and forehead. This higher humming is said to be very beneficial for the pituitary gland.

34. Practice Tratak meditation as a daily practice. Light a candle and use the candle flame to focus the eyes. Apart from calming the mind it stimulates the pituitary and pineal glands

35. Sleep in complete darkness so your body produces more melatonin. For instance, your bedside clock might emit too much light

Bibliography

Online references

http://www.etymonline.com
http://www.merriam-webster.com/
http://www.bachcenter.com/center/remedies.htm
http://www.louisehay.com/about-louise/
http://www.religionfacts.com/a-z-religion-index/deepak
_chopra.htm

Book References

Schuessler, Dr. W. H., Handbook of the Biochemic Tissue Salts, (1991), Australia, Martin & Pleasance

Ponder, C., *The Healing Secret of the Ages Revealed,* (1966), New York, Parker Publishing Co. Inc

Bach, E., *The Twelve Healers and other Remedies,* (1936), London, CW Daniel

Tansley, David, V., *Radionics and the Subtle Anatomy of Man*, (1998), New York, Beekman Pub

Blavatsky's, H. P., The *Secret Doctrine,* (2010), Nabu Press

Stanley Alder, V., *The Fifth Dimensions,* (2000), UK, Weiser Books

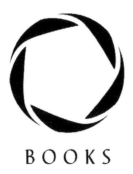

BOOKS

O is a symbol of the world, of oneness and unity. In different cultures it also means the "eye," symbolizing knowledge and insight. We aim to publish books that are accessible, constructive and that challenge accepted opinion, both that of academia and the "moral majority."

Our books are available in all good English language bookstores worldwide. If you don't see the book on the shelves ask the bookstore to order it for you, quoting the ISBN number and title. Alternatively you can order online (all major online retail sites carry our titles) or contact the distributor in the relevant country, listed on the copyright page.

See our website **www.o-books.net** for a full list of over 500 titles, growing by 100 a year.

And tune in to myspiritradio.com for our book review radio show, hosted by June-Elleni Laine, where you can listen to the authors discussing their books.

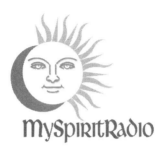

Printed and bound by CPI Group (UK) Ltd, Croydon, CR0 4YY

14/01/2025

01820090-0002